S/NVQ level 1

introducing hairdressing

2nd edition

Christine McMillan–Bodell

www.harcourt.co.uk

✓ Free online support
✓ Useful weblinks
✓ 24 hour online ordering

01865 888058

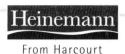

Heinemann

From Harcourt

Heinemann Educational Publishers
Halley Court, Jordan Hill, Oxford OX2 8EJ
Part of Harcourt Education

Heinemann is the registered trademark of Harcourt Education Limited

Text © Christine McMillan-Bodell, 2004

This edition first published 2007
First edition published 2004

10 09 08 07
10 9 8 7 6 5 4 3 2 1

British Library Cataloguing in Publication Data is available from the British Library on request.

10-digit ISBN: 0 435 46466 3
13-digit ISBN: 978 0 435464 66 0

Designed by Tower Designs UK Limited

Typeset by Tower Designs UK Limited

Original illustrations © Harcourt Education Limited, 2006

Illustrated by Eikon Ltd., Kamae Design Limited and Tower Designs UK Limited

Cover design by David Poole

Printed by South China Printing Co Ltd

Cover photo © Corbis

Acknowledgements

Every effort has been made to contact copyright holders of material reproduced in this book. Any omissions will be rectified in subsequent printings if notice is given to the publishers.

Without the never-ending love, support and 100 per cent commitment of my immediate family, loved one and friends, this book certainly would never have been written.

My thanks are also extended to my colleague Sylvia Stephenson for her valuable expertise in African-Caribbean hairdressing.

Thank you to Aylesbury Buckinghamshire College, for its assistance in facilitating the photo shoot, together with their students, models and staff.

Thank you to Jules Selmes, our professional photographer, who worked us all very hard during the photo shoot.

Finally, to all at Heinemann – editor, artists, researchers – thank you, for what I never dreamed possible.

Christine McMillan-Bodell

Use of HABIA unit titles and element headings by kind permission of HABIA, Fraser House, Nether Hall Road, Doncaster, South Yorkshire, DN1 2PH, Tel: 01302 380028, Email: enquiries@habia.org.uk, Website: www.habia.org.uk.

The author and publisher would like to thank the following for permission to reproduce photographs: Gareth Boden – pages 5, 72, 73, 87, 109; Getty Images / Stone – page 1; Harcourt Education Ltd. / Tudor Photography – 82, 110, 111; Chris Honeywell – all other photos; iStockPhoto / Heidi Anglesey – page 7; Masterfile / Robert Karpa – page 9; Masterfile / Anthony Redpath – page 62; Photos.com – page 67; Rex Features / Heptagon – 38; Science Photo Library – pages 84, 85; Jules Selmes – 12, 17, 19, 20, 24, 26, 31, 39, 51, 52, 54, 58, 64, 76, 100

Contents

Introduction

Why hairdressing?

If you are interested in hairdressing as a career, then read on...

The hairdressing industry is a multi-billion pound industry. It employs more than 203,000 people in the UK. There is a growing demand for skilled hairdressers as more and more of us realise that a healthy lifestyle involves keeping fit and looking good.

Today's hairdressers cater for the needs of a multi-ethnic society – from European to Asian to African-Caribbean. There is also a vast range of products available to both you as a hairdresser and to your client, including the latest organically formulated treatments.

Once you are a highly skilled hairdresser, there's an exciting future waiting for you in a high-tech industry, with the chance to become your own boss, enjoy job security and travel the world.

About this book

Introducing Hairdressing will introduce you to NVQ1 and the basics of hairdressing. The book has been written to the 2003 standards. It covers all of the relevant performance criteria and range statements linked to NVQ1 Hairdressing.

The book looks at both African-Caribbean and European hairdressing and includes illustrated step-by-step guides to help you learn practical hairdressing procedures. The introductory unit, 'All about hair', covers what you will need to know about the structure of hair and hair types.

To help you achieve each unit of work, the book contains:

- 'check it out' questions linked to NVQ1 performance criteria and range statements
- 'chat room' features designed to help you think about the practicalities of hairdressing and the type of situations you will have to deal with every day
- 'think about it' questions that will help you to develop your job role
- memory joggers at the end of each unit which will help you to reflect on what you have learned
- word searches.

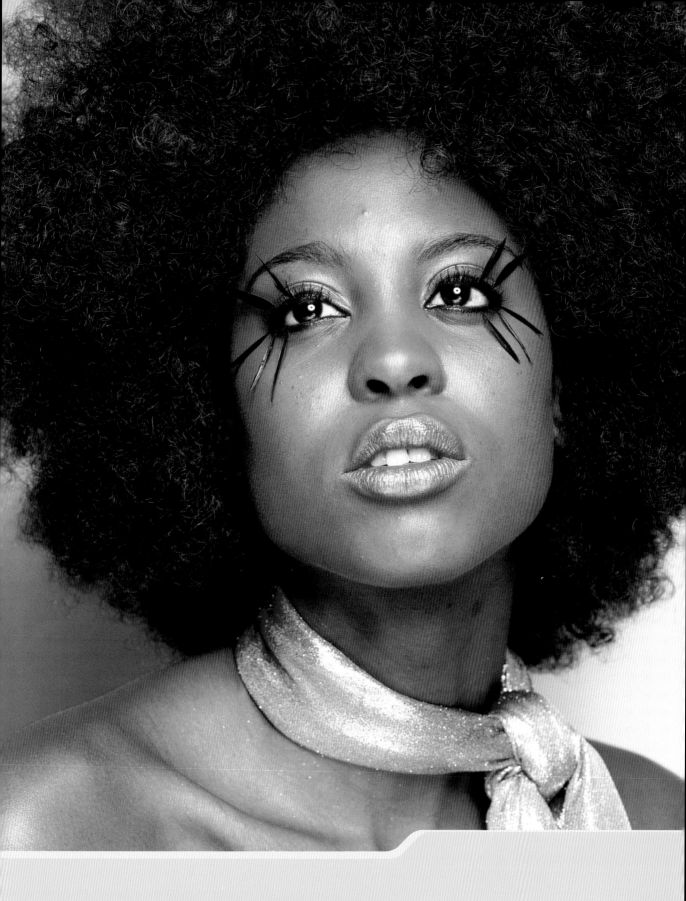

ABOUT HAIR

Why do you have hair?

For protection

Hair helps to protect you. If an object were to fall on your head, the hair on your scalp would give you some protection. The hair inside your nose acts as a filter when breathing. It helps to prevent dust and debris from entering your nasal passages. Your eyelashes also help to prevent dust entering your eyes.

For warmth

Hair acts as an insulator – it helps to keep the surface of the skin warm. You may have noticed the hairs on your skin standing up when you are cold. This is how the body tries to keep you warm, by trapping a layer of warm air between the surface of the skin and the hair.

To help you look good

How does your hair make you feel? Mostly, when your hair looks good, you are likely to feel good. A freshly shampooed and well-conditioned head of hair is likely to give you added confidence. Your hair acts as a frame around your face rather like a frame around a painting. Your hair can be styled to suit your face shape and perhaps to disguise a less-than-attractive feature.

The hair's structure

Let's look at the basic structure of hair. Hair is made of a protein called keratin. Your skin and nails are also made from this protein.

The hair shaft has three layers:

- the cuticle

- the cortex

- the medulla.

The three main layers of the hair shaft

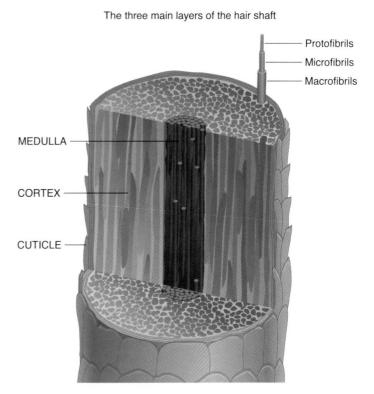

Protofibrils
Microfibrils
Macrofibrils

MEDULLA

CORTEX

CUTICLE

The hair shaft

CHAT ROOM

The goodness you get from the food that you eat is used to make the basic building blocks of your body – amino acids. These link together to make keratin. Think about what you eat and its effect on your hair. Hair loss and scalp problems can be caused by a poor diet.

The cuticle

The outer layer of the hair shaft is called the cuticle. It is made of overlapping scales which are wrapped around the centre of the hair (known as the cortex). The cuticle scales knit together tightly giving the hair shaft a **non-porous** outer layer.

Non-porous – does not allow liquid or air through.

When hair is in good condition the scales lie flat and reflect the light. The hair looks smooth and shiny.

The cortex

The cortex layer of the hair shaft is made up of bundles of fibrils. Imagine holding a bundle of dried spaghetti in your hand – this will give you a good idea of what the cortex layer looks like.

THINK ABOUT IT

Think of examples of porous and non-porous substances.

Chemical treatments such as perming, relaxing, straightening, bleaching and permanent colouring alter the basic structure of the hair shaft. This takes place in the cortex.

The medulla

The central layer of the hair is the medulla. It has no part to play in hairdressing. It is simply made up of air spaces along the length of the hair shaft. The medulla may be present in some hairs, but not in others, and may not be present for the full length of the hair.

Hair condition, length and hair types

Hair condition

Hair and scalp conditions can be split into:

- dry
- normal
- greasy
- dandruff affected.

Hair in good condition

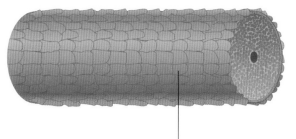

Cuticle scales lying close together

Hair in bad condition

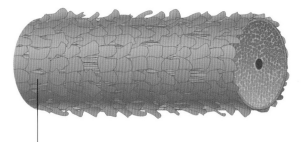

Cuticle scales open and mishapen. Some scales may
have been completely destroyed, exposing the cortex

Hair in good condition is soft to touch while hair in poor condition
feels rough, dry and brittle.

*Hair in good and
poor condition*

Length

The length of hair will help you to decide how you should shampoo
it. For example, hair above or below the shoulders may need a front
or backwash shampoo.

Types of hair

The differences between Caucasian/European, African-Caribbean and
Asian/Oriental hair are important when choosing the most
appropriate shampoo.

- The Caucasian/European hair shaft can be straight, wavy or curly
  and is oval shaped.
- The African-Caribbean hair shaft can be tightly or loosely curled
  and is kidney shaped.
- The Asian hair shaft can be straight and/or coarse and is round
  in shape.

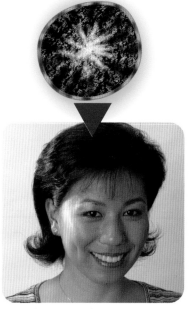

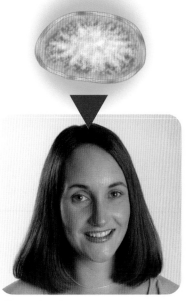

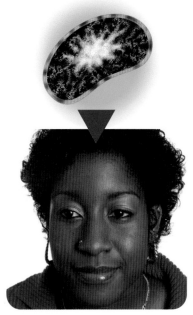

Asian hair   *Caucasian/European hair*   *African-Caribbean hair*

Cross sections of hair shafts for different types of hair

The texture of hair will vary from client to client and may also vary within the same head of hair. Texture can be fine, medium or coarse, with fine-textured hair having a small circumference and coarse-textured hair having a large circumference. To find out the texture, run your fingers along the length of a single hair. This information will be useful when you are choosing products to apply to the client's hair and scalp.

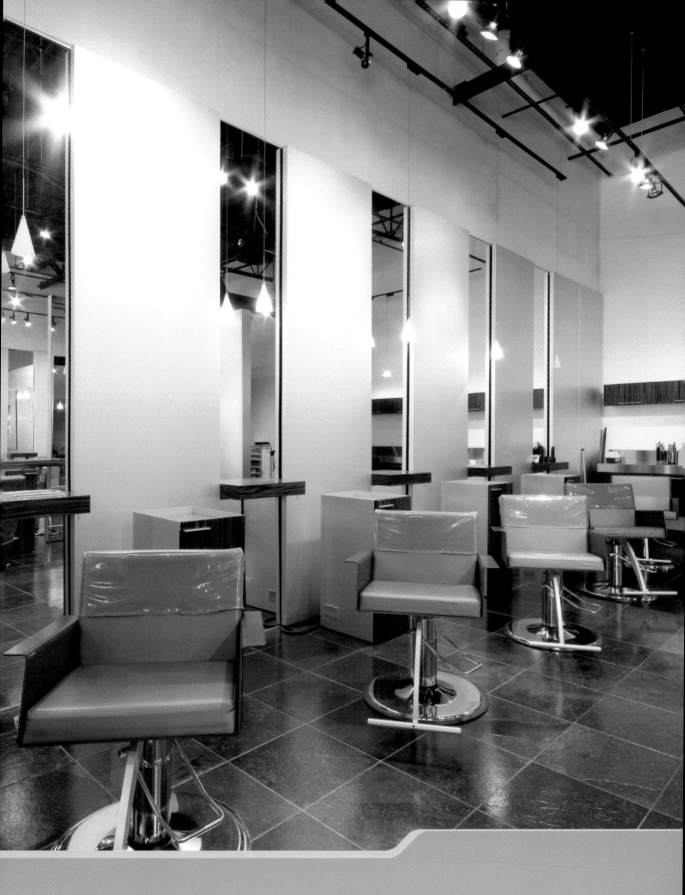

IN THE WORKPLACE

Hairdressing is a thriving, fun-loving, people-oriented industry and you need to follow certain procedures when you're working with electrical equipment, chemical substances and the public. Health and safety should be observed in three key areas:

- your employer's responsibilities to you, your colleagues, clients and visitors
- your responsibility to your colleagues and yourself
- and your responsibility to your clients.

This unit covers the health and safety duties for everyone in the hairdressing industry and it relates directly to the current HABIA (Hair and Beauty Industry Authority) occupational standards for hairdressing. In this unit you will learn:

- how to identify the hazards and evaluate the risks in your workplace
- who is responsible for health and safety at work
- which health and safety policies relate to you
- about the most appropriate fire-fighting equipment for use in your salon
- how to reduce the risks to health and safety in your workplace
- about any harmful practices in your salon.

The salon is a great place to work, however you must be aware of risks and hazards

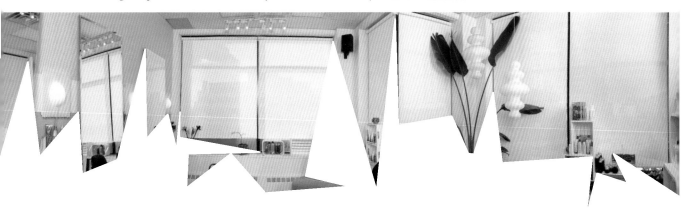

Identify the hazards and evaluate the risks in your workplace

Attention to health and safety is as much a part of customer service as good communication, and is an indicator of your professionalism. At the most basic level, you would think again about going back to a stylist who used dirty brushes in an untidy and neglected salon – no matter how brilliant the cut and colour.

This unit covers the health and safety duties for everyone in the hairdressing industry. Every employee and employer is required to behave safely and professionally. You must always be responsible for your own behaviour and make sure that your actions do not create a health and safety risk. For example, if you see something in the salon that is potentially dangerous you must take sensible action towards putting things right. This may involve writing the risk down and/or reporting it to a more senior member of staff.

You need to demonstrate that you understand the health and safety requirements and policies in the salon. You should be constantly improving your own working practices and work areas, preventing any risk of you or others being harmed. You must be able to identify risks arising from any hazards you have identified. You must know which risks you can deal with safely within the limits of your own authority, and which risks must be reported to a more senior member of staff.

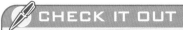

CHECK IT OUT

Who is this senior member of staff within your salon?

Evidence is important when creating your portfolio. You must provide examples of how you have taken steps to reduce health and safety risks.

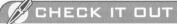

CHECK IT OUT

Draw a simple plan of the hairdressing salon where you work. Use a key to indicate on the plan where the fire exits, specified assembly points, fire extinguishers and first aid equipment are located.

'Get smart, get trained and get it right, first time, every time'

The **Health and Safety at Work Act (1974)**, covers everyone in the salon – employees, self-employed people and visitors, such as technical reps and clients. You must be trained before you carry out any job within the salon – no matter how small or how quick the task is. Professional hairdressers are legally bound to abide by manufacturers' instructions, the salon policy and local bylaws.

Failure to abide by the Act can result in heavy penalties. Criminal proceedings, heavy fines and/or imprisonment do happen – not just for salon owners, but also for the individual responsible for failing to comply. If you have any issues about health and safety, discuss these with a member of staff. Make sure that the discussion is recorded, and that any action required is followed up. In this unit you will learn about a variety of policies and regulations that you must follow during your working life.

 CHECK IT OUT

Alan had been working in the hairdressing salon each Saturday for three months. The salon owner had been keen to advance Alan's knowledge and often demonstrated hairdressing techniques to him. This included removing colours, shampooing and rinsing perms. Alan was responsible for the usual day-to-day duties, such as client care and general salon organisation. One Saturday near Christmas Alan had a lot of clients to deal with. He was asked to place a plastic cap over a client's bleached hair and place her under a dryer.

Alan had been keen to learn the correct way to apply and process bleach and always read the manufacturers' instructions. He discovered that dry heat was not recommended for this type of bleach and quietly explained this to the stylist. At this time the client started to complain that she was uncomfortable under the hood dryer. Alan went to investigate and discovered that the bleach had run down the client's neck and back, bleaching her clothes and burning her skin. Alan was then instructed to rinse the client's hair and deal with her clothes as best as he could. The client was angry that no apology was offered by the stylist and claimed that she would sue.

Who is negligent? Can the client sue both Alan and the salon owner? Discuss this situation with your colleagues.

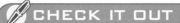**CHECK IT OUT**

Verbally and non-verbally, report any hazard to a senior member of staff, and provide evidence that you have dealt with hazards that present a risk.

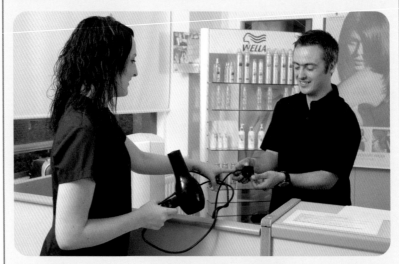

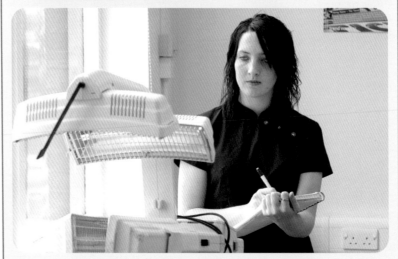

If you find faulty equipment report it to a senior colleague and make a note of the discussion

Risks and hazards

Your work role includes carrying out duties safely in accordance with manufacturers' instructions, local bylaws and salon policy. You have a legal duty to reduce the risks and hazards in your workplace.

A **hazard** is something that could cause harm.

A **risk** is the likelihood of the hazard causing harm.

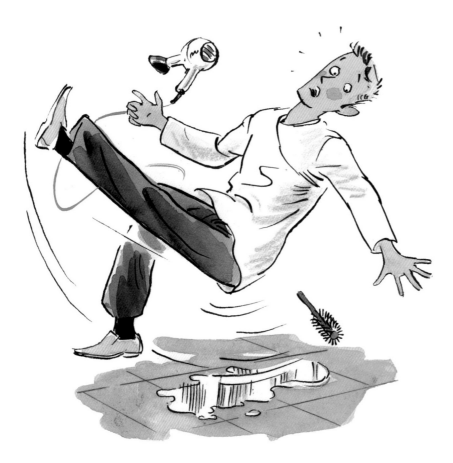

Slippery surfaces present a risk to you and your clients

 CHECK IT OUT

After reading the following paragraphs, make a list of the potentially harmful working practices that you come into contact with on a daily basis.

Within the salon you must identify working practices which could harm yourself or other people. Remaining alert to potential hazards will help protect everyone in the salon at any time. Remember that you need to concentrate and keep alert when dealing with products, tools and equipment.

Your physical wellbeing is essential not only to yourself but also to others within the salon. Too many late nights, over indulgence in food or alcohol, or additional stress with personal issues will all have a bearing on how you carry out your day-to-day duties. Be mindful that you are part of a team – if one person does not give 100 per cent it will have a serious impact on the health and safety of the team and your clients.

 THINK ABOUT IT

What does the word hazard mean?

See if you can give two examples of hazards and two examples of risks in the salon.

Describe your responsibilities for health and safety in the salon as an employee.

Because you will often rely on the use of electrical equipment in the salon you should pay particular attention to The Electricity at Work Regulations (1989). We need to be careful prior to using pieces of equipment in order that we minimise the risk of accidents to both our clients and ourselves.

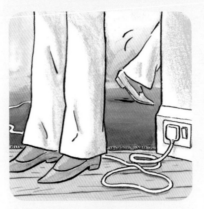

*A trailing cable from a hairdryer is a **hazard**. If it is allowed to cross over a walkway, it may cause an accident.*

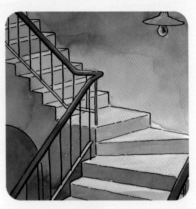

*A failed light bulb is a hazard. It may be only a low **risk** if the work area is well lit, but a high risk if it lights up a set of steps.*

Hazard – *something with the potential to cause harm.*

Risk – *the likelihood that a hazard will cause harm.*

Have a look at the following documentation and complete it with the help of a colleague. When complete, check the details with a senior member of staff.

HAZARD CHECKLIST
Which hazards are present in my workplace?

Date ....   Checked by ....

	Relevant to my workplace?	Risk assessment complete?
Fire		
Electric shock		
Posture		
Workplace environmental conditions		
Use of mains gas appliances		
Use and storage of chemical substances		
Hazardous substances		
Slips and trips		
Falls		
Falling objects		
Stress		
Work equipment		
Maintenance		
Infection control		
Other (list)		

Health and safety laws

We are now going to look at the key factors within each of the health and safety laws that affect you within your day-to-day work. The acts that you should be aware of are listed below.

- The Fire Precautions Act (1971)
- The Health and Safety at Work Act (1974)
- The Electricity at Work Regulations (1989)
- The Workplace (Health, Safety and Welfare) Regulations (1992)
- The Manual Handling Operations Regulations (1992)
- The Personal Protective Equipment (PPE) at Work Regulations (1992)
- The Reporting of Injuries, Diseases and Dangerous Occurrences Regulations (RIDDOR) (1995)
- The Provision and Use of Work Equipment at Work Regulations (1998)
- The Control of Substances Hazardous to Health Regulations (COSHH) (2002)

The Fire Precautions Act (1971)

If you discover a fire you must raise the alarm calmly and safely. Staff, clients and visitors must be notified and escorted from the building using the nearest fire exit.

Dial 999 and ask the operator for the fire service. Give the operator your name and the address of the salon, as well as brief details of the situation that they are likely to be involved in.

If you have been trained in fire fighting – and if the fire is small – use the most appropriate fire extinguisher to tackle the fire – but only if it is safe for you to do so.

Under the Fire Precautions Act (1971) all premises are required to have fire-fighting equipment, which must be maintained in good working order.

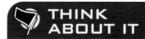

THINK ABOUT IT

Evidence is important when creating your portfolio and within your own work role. Provide some examples a how you have taken steps to reduce health and safety risks in the salon.

CHECK IT OUT

Find out where your fire-fighting equipment is in the salon.

How often do you have a fire drill?

What types of fire extinguisher do you have?

Fire is dangerous – if you discover a fire you should treat it with caution. Breathing in hot air from a fire can damage your airways and lungs. Burning chemicals can give off toxic fumes; if you breathe these they can cause asphyxiation. Smoke-filled buildings are a health hazard because you cannot see or breathe.

Fire can damage the salon by causing decorations to smoulder, ceilings to collapse, fixtures and fittings to burn and damage to walls. Fire damage to the salon can lead to blocked passageways, which could cause a lethal hazard – someone could suffocate due to a lack of oxygen.

To put out a fire you need to be trained in dealing with a variety of different fires. You can be trained to use a fire extinguisher in order to put out *small* fires. To extinguish a fire you need to remove one of its three components – oxygen, heat or fuel.

Types of fire extinguisher

There are many ways in which to put fires out safely and we must remember that the fire extinguishers provided in the salon are there for a professional purpose. All fire extinguishers are colour coded to indicate the type of fire that the fire extinguisher can be used for.

THINK ABOUT IT

A fire needs three main components:
- fuel
- oxygen
- and heat.

What could you use to remove the oxygen?

What could you use to remove the heat?

What could you use to remove the fuel?

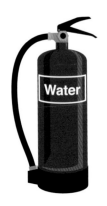 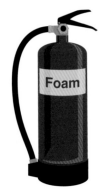 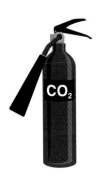 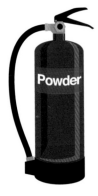 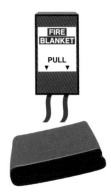

Class A	*Class B*	*Class C*	*Class Electrical*	*Class F*
A water extinguisher can be used to put out fires involving paper, coal, textiles and wood.	*A foam extinguisher can be used to put out fires involving flammable liquids such as grease, oil, petrol and paints (but not cooking oil or grease).*	*A carbon dioxide extinguisher can be used to put out fires involving flammable gases.*	*A dry powder extinguisher can be used to put out electrical fires.*	*A blanket can be used to put out fires involving cooking oils and fats.*

REMEMBER!
Knowing which types of extinguisher should never be used on which types of fire is as important as knowing which types of extinguisher should be used on which types of fire.

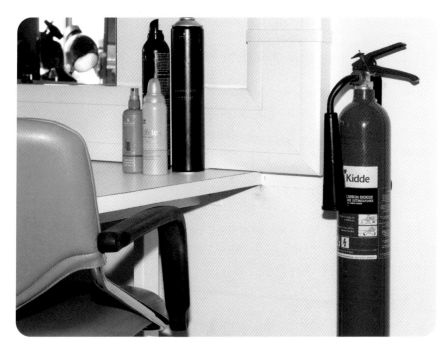

Fire extinguishers should be easily accessible

Many fires could be avoided if simple house-keeping rules were applied in the workplace.

- Fire doors must be kept closed and unlocked to prevent the fire from spreading and to enable staff and visitors to leave the buildings safely.
- Keep fire exits free from rubbish at all times.
- All electrical equipment must be used in accordance with the manufacturers' instructions and must be regularly inspected by a qualified electrician.
- Correct fuses must be fitted and sockets must not be overloaded.
- Keep aerosols away from any heat source – including the sun and radiators.
- Carelessness causes fires – look out for your own and others' safety.

The Health and Safety at Work Act (1974)

The Health and Safety at Work Act (1974) covers everyone – employees, self-employed people and visitors, such as technical reps and clients. The Act covers a variety of working practices and is linked to many associated pieces of legislation covering any specific job role within any industry. The Act informs both employer and employee with respect to many aspects of health and safety within the workplace and outlines everybody's duties and responsibilities. Employers have slightly different obligations from employees.

> ### THINK ABOUT IT
>
> Which types of fire extinguisher can be used on more than one fire?
>
> Which types of fire extinguisher should never be used on which types of fire?

Employers are bound by a duty of care to each of their employees. This means that everything that an employer does when setting up and running a business will be done with the safety of all who come into contact with the business in mind. In order for this to be effective, the following must be adhered to by all employers:

■ a workplace and systems of work must be provided and maintained

■ the use, handling, storage and transport of articles and substances must be accounted for

■ information, instruction, training and supervision must be provided

■ access and exits must be clear and free from hazard

■ the working environment, facilities and welfare arrangements must comply with the Act.

The Act's key message

It is your duty to maintain the health and safety of yourself and others who may be affected by your actions.

CHECK IT OUT

Create a tree diagram of the staff in your salon, starting at the top with the salon owner and working down. Indicate each person's name, job title and their responsibilities. Identify the person who is responsible for reporting any accidents to the health and safety executive.

The Electricity at Work Regulations (1989)

A qualified electrician must test every electrical appliance in the salon once a year. This includes 'domestic' equipment, such as the washing machine, the fridge, the cooker, and the kettle, as well as all of the specific hairdressing equipment. A written record must be kept of these tests and shown to the health and safety authorities upon inspection.

The Act's key message

All electrical equipment must be used appropriately and with precaution, checked and tested. The position of plugs and sockets must be safe and the space you are working in must have adequate lighting. Any faulty or damaged equipment must be removed from use, labelled and reported to a responsible person.

Safe use and storage of electrical equipment

All salons depend on electrical equipment such as hand-held hairdryers and steamers, so it is important to handle and store equipment safely. Below are some guidelines on the safe use and storage of electrical equipment.

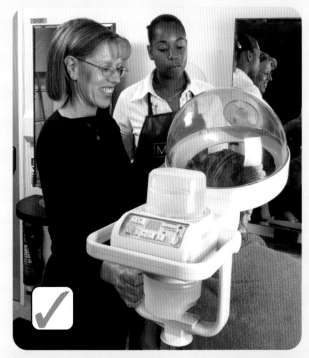

Know how to use the equipment.

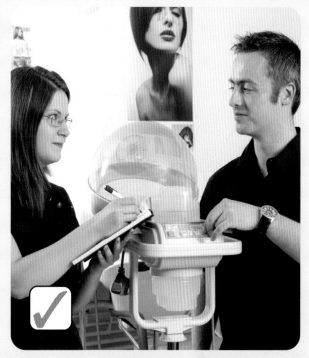

Be trained in the equipment's use.

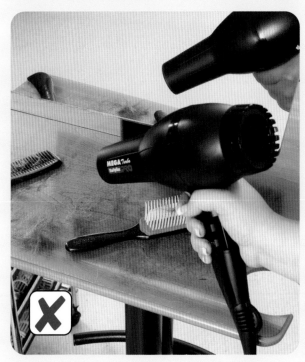

Use the equipment only for the purpose intended.

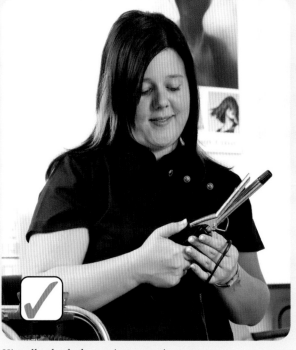

Visually check the equipment prior to use.

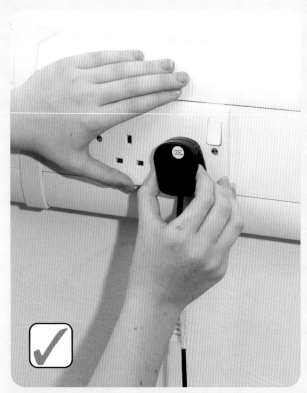

Switch off the equipment and remove from the power supply when finished.

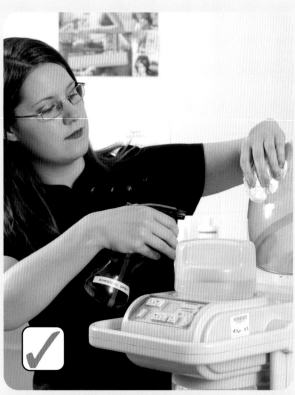

Clean the equipment after each use.

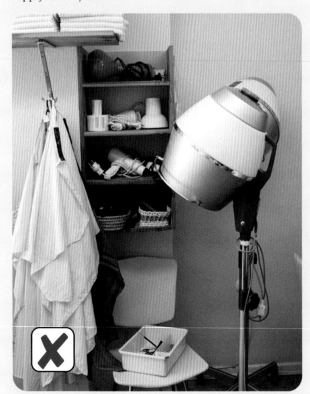

Store the equipment safely, in an allocated area.

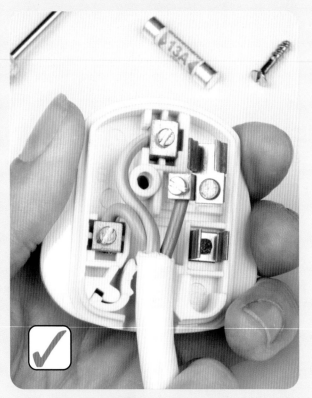

Test the equipment regularly – this should be carried out by a qualified electrician.

The Workplace (Health, Safety and Welfare) Regulations (1992)

This regulation requires all at work to help maintain a safe and healthy working environment. Every employer is required to provide a safe working environment for all at work.

The Act's key message

When working in the salon you must maintain a safe and healthy environment.

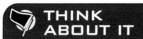

THINK ABOUT IT

Think about your responsibilities in your job. Read the list of workplace regulations and write a simple statement about how each point affects you in your day-to-day work in the salon.

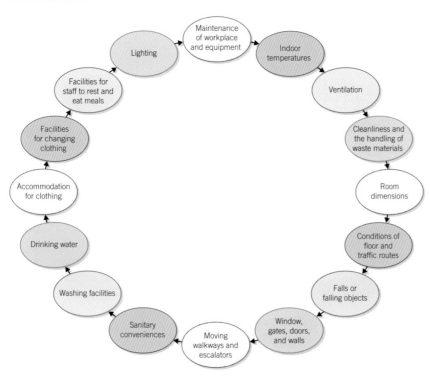

The Manual Handling Operations Regulations (1992)

This Act requires certain measures, such as following a set way of dealing with heavy or awkward-shaped deliveries. The Act deals with lifting items, pushing or pulling hairdressing trolleys, carrying loads and stacking shelves. All people at work must minimise the risks from lifting and handling objects.

CHECK IT OUT

Write a simple list of the different working practices that you come across. It may be that all of these practices are carried out differently in your salon. Discuss your findings with your colleagues.

The Act's key message

This Act provides guidelines for protecting yourself and others whilst minimising risks when lifting heavy objects.

Safe handling practices when dealing with hazards and risks

A box of heavy stock is an example of a hazard – it presents a risk to someone who needs to lift it manually, so safe-handling practices must be adopted. The most common types of injury from an incorrect lift are back strain and pulled muscles.

Assess the risk

Assess the box before you attempt to move it. Is it too heavy or bulky to move safely? If so, you could empty part of the order before lifting, or ask another member of staff for help.

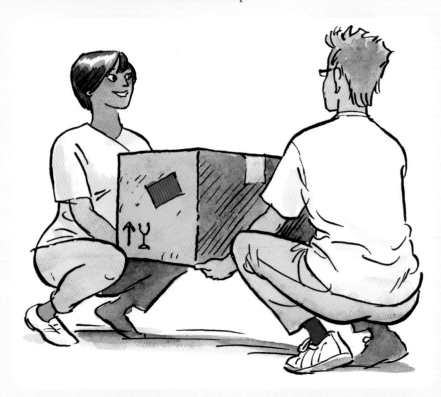

If something is too heavy for you to carry on your own, ask a colleague for help

You must be trained in correct lifting practice, as with all aspects of your day-to-day work. Plan your route and remove any obstructions. Do you have a safe passageway to carry this load? Where are you going to store it? Think about the lift that you are planning. Is the load to be lifted of a regular shape? Does it have sharp edges? Do you need to wear protective gloves? Are you wearing suitable clothes that will allow you to bend and move freely?

Safe lifting practices

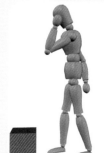 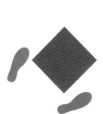 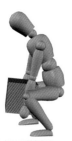 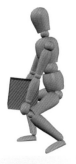 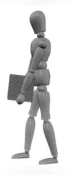 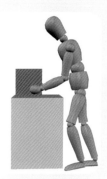

1 Think about the lift. Where is the load to be placed? Do you need help? Are handling aids available?

2 Get ready to lift. Stand with your feet apart.

3 Bend your knees. Keep your back straight. Tuck in your chin. Lean slightly forward over the load to get a good grip.

4 Get a good grip on the load and lift smoothly.

5 Carry the load at waist height to keep a low centre of gravity.

6 Set the object down carefully.

1 Check that you're wearing appropriate clothes. Are your shoes sensible? Is your movement unrestricted?

2 Stand with your feet apart, your weight should be evenly spread over both feet.

3 Bend your knees slowly, keeping your back straight. Tuck your chin in towards your chest. Get a good grip on the base of the box.

4 Bring the load up to your waist height, keeping the lift as smooth as possible.

5 Keep the box close to your body. Proceed carefully making sure that you can see where you are going.

6 Lower the load, reversing the lifting procedure.

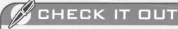

CHECK IT OUT

Watch people lift objects from the floor. Do they bend from the hips or do they bend from the knees? How should they bend?

The Personal Protective Equipment at Work Regulations (1992)

PPE – *Personal Protective Equipment.*

The Personal Protective Equipment (**PPE**) legislation states that you must wear suitable protective gloves and an apron when dealing with any chemical or harmful substance linked with chemical treatments. You must always wear PPE when working with chemical substances and clients must be suitably protected during the chemical treatment.

By ensuring your use of personal protective equipment, you will meet the health and safety regulations and workplace policies. Remember that PPE includes preparing your clients' hair and protecting their skin where necessary prior to any chemical treatment.

The Act's key message

Your employer must provide appropriate personal protective equipment for working with chemical treatments and you must always use it when applicable.

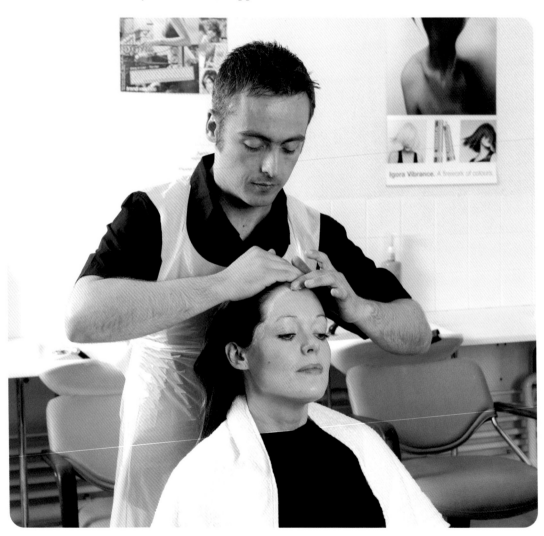

Personal protective equipment must be worn when working with chemical treatments

The Reporting of Injuries, Diseases and Dangerous Occurrences Regulations (RIDDOR) (1995)

All injuries must be reported to the member of staff responsible for health and safety. The salon accident book must be completed with basic personal details of the person (or people) involved and a detailed description of the incident. Because there might be legal consequences due to the injury, all witnesses must provide clear and accurate details of what happened.

The Act's key message

You must report:

- fatal accidents
- any major injury sustained at work
- work-related diseases
- any potentially dangerous event that takes place at work
- accidents causing more than three days' absence from work.

The Provision and Use of Work Equipment at Work Regulations (1998)

These regulations lay down important health and safety controls on the provision and use of work equipment. Employers must provide equipment for use that is properly constructed, suitable for its purpose and kept in good working order. Training on how to use each piece of equipment must be provided by the employer. Staff who use the salon equipment must be competent in its use.

The Act's key message

You must be competent when using tools and equipment in the salon.

The Control of Substances Hazardous to Health (COSHH) Regulations (2002)

Chemicals, including perm lotions, neutralisers and hydrogen peroxide, are hazardous and present a high risk. They must be handled, stored, used and disposed of correctly in accordance with COSHH 2002. This means that every chemical and product used within the salon must be assessed for risk.

Find out about the working practices within your salon and those which are relevant to your own job description. It's easy to forget the risks involved in using shampoos and conditioners; remember that the ingredients can cause skin and scalp irritation. All manufacturers are duty-bound to inform you of the ingredients in each hairdressing product stored in your salon. Each item must be catalogued in a register for staff to access so that all staff are trained to deal with the possible dangers of the products that they use.

Many products, such as hairspray, mousse, perm lotion and hydrogen peroxide, are potentially hazardous and should be stored in a cool, dark, locked fire-proof cabinet – preferably on a low shelf.

Potentially hazardous products should be stored in a locked cabinet

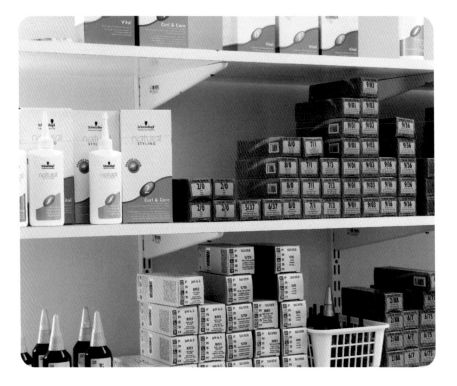

Reading and following manufacturers' instructions must support any duty that is carried out in the salon. You must use products, tools and equipment for their intended purpose. Thoroughly sterilise all tools and equipment and maintain a healthy and safe environment. This will help you make the correct decision when using products on your clients and choosing the correct equipment for the treatment they are about to receive. The client can then have the added confidence that you have considered all possible options and that the products and equipment will be used safely and hygienically.

The Act's key message

Any substances in use in your salon that could be hazardous to health should be stored, handled, used and disposed of according to legislation, manufacturers' instructions and local bylaws.

A Guide to the Health and Safety Salon Hair Products

Hair preparations should not present a risk to the health and safety of hairdressers or their clients if used sensibly and manufacturers instructions are followed.

The purpose of this booklet is to provide sufficient information on the HAIR PRODUCTS used in salons, for you to make an assessment as required by the COSHH Regulations.

Use MUST also be made of the product lists issued by manufacturers which specify the section in the booklet to which each of their products refer.

It should be noted that this booklet only covers products marketed by the companies listed on page 5.

The information given in this booklet is ONLY PART of what is required to meet the assessment requirements of COSHH. Information will be also required on any other products used in the salon which may be hazardous to health, such as those used for cleaning and disinfection.

The Health & Safety Executive (HSE) has been consulted during the preparation of this booklet and their comments have been incorporated.

Keep a copy of this booklet in the salon for reference purposes and for discussion with your local authority inspector.

HYDROGEN PEROXIDE SOLUTION

Composition
Stabilised acidic aqueous solutions or emulsions containing hydrogen peroxide of various strengths for use with:

Permanent Colorants
Bleach powder
Permanent waves as neutralisers

Ingredients
Hydrogen peroxide
Hair tighteners Colorant remover up to 40 vol or 12%
Preparations containing higher concentrations of hydrogen peroxide are outside the scope of the Cosmetics Directive. In such cases, seek the advice of the supplier regarding COSHH assessments.

Hazards Identification
Irritant to eyes and skin.

First-Aid Measures
Eyes: Rinse eyes immediately with plenty of water. If irritation persists seek medical advice.
Skin: Wash skin immediately with water. If irritation persists seek medical advice.
Ingestion: Seek medical advice immediately.

Accidental release measures
Always use water to dilute and mop up spillages.

Handling & Storage
Always use non-metallic utensils to avoid rapid decomposition of the product. Do not allow contact with easily combustible materials such as paper. Store in cool, dry place away from sunlight and other sources of heat. Always store hydrogen peroxide in the container supplied. It is particularly important that no contamination enters the containers as this could lead to decomposition resulting in the liberation of heat and oxygen. Therefore, replace cap immediately after use.

Exposure Controls/Personal Protection
Always wear suitable protective gloves. Avoid contact with eyes and face. Do not use on abraded or sensitive skin.

Stability & Reactivity
Hydrogen peroxide may react with other chemicals to form dangerous materials (e.g. explosive). Therefore, avoid mixtures other than recognised formulations. Combustion may occur if hydrogen peroxide is allowed to dry out on materials such as paper, hair, wood etc.

Disposal
Wash down the drain with plenty of water. Do not incinerate.

REMEMBER!
Good ventilation is important when mixing colours and bleaches and when using colouring preparations. Windows and/or an air vent must be opened, as chemicals can be dangerous if inhaled.

MEMORY JOGGER

1. Think of three safe practices when using colouring and bleaching products.

2. What effect could unprofessional behaviour have on your colleagues and clients?

3. What does COSHH mean?

4. Describe your responsibilities for health and safety as an employee in the salon.

5. Who is the person responsible for reporting health and safety matters in the salon?

6. To whom would you report the following risks?

   ▪ An electrical socket that has too many pieces of equipment plugged into it

   ▪ A damaged fire extinguisher

   ▪ A blocked fire exit

   ▪ A chemical spillage

Workplace policies

If there are more than five people employed in your salon, a workplace policy is required. The policy is written to clarify what the risks are at work on a day-to-day basis, to bring to your attention any precautions that may be necessary and to clarify who is responsible for what.

All members of staff must co-operate with the workplace policy to make sure that the salon is a safe and healthy place to work. This should include checking that work areas are kept clean, fire exits aren't blocked and that you have enough space to work comfortably without bumping into workstations or other salon staff.

 CHECK IT OUT

Find out if the salon where you work has a workplace policy.

Design a simple chart with the names of the staff who are responsible and what they are responsible for in terms of health and safety.

Do you have a member of staff who is qualified as a first aider?

What happens in the salon when the first aider is absent?

How would you contact the first aider? Is their phone number in the staff room or in reception?

Sterilising equipment

The importance of sterilising your tools is paramount to a hygienic working environment and will promote a high standard of cleanliness to your clients and colleagues and prevent the risk of cross-infection and infestation. Remember that you must clean your equipment before using any sterilising method. Only tools and equipment that have been cleaned can be thoroughly sterilised.

The methods of sterilisation available in the salon may include:
- barbicide
- ultraviolet
- autoclave.

You must use tools and equipment that are clean, safe and fit for their purpose – tools and equipment identified at the time of consultation must be readily available to use for professional purposes. This includes pintail combs to weave sections of hair, highlighting hooks to pull strands of hair through a highlighting cap, professional foil strips to assist colouring, etc. Equipment should be cleaned and sterilised as soon after use as is practical to ensure that it is ready for the next treatment.

Barbicide

The most popular method of sterilising is barbicide. Barbicide is quick and easy to use, but will only inhibit the growth of bacteria. You must read and follow the manufacturers' instructions when making up the solution and you must remember to change it daily.

Ultraviolet

Placing tools that are clean and dry in an ultraviolet cabinet will prevent the growth of bacteria. You must remember to turn your tools over every 15 minutes to keep both sides hygienically clean.

Autoclave

The most successful method of sterilising is the autoclave, which will completely destroy all living bacteria on the surface of your tools. However, not all equipment can withstand the heat of an autoclave – this sterilises at up to 125°C!

Are your salon practices safe?

Find out if there are any differences between workplace policies and suppliers' or manufacturers' instructions in relation to day-to-day practical jobs. Think about neutralising, rinsing off a colour and blow-drying your client's hair. These are practical activities, which are carried out every day in every salon and you will find that practices vary.

MEMORY JOGGER

How would you deal with the following?
(a) Faulty electrical equipment
(b) Slippery surfaces

Why should you remain alert to the presence of hazards?

What could happen if there were obstructions to the entry and exit doors of your salon?

Public- and treatment-liability insurance

Did you know that all salons are duty-bound to take out public- and treatment-liability insurance?

If a member of staff were to injure one of your clients in the salon as a result of negligence, the client would have grounds to sue the member of staff and the salon.

The employer's insurance certificate must cover all staff, clients and visitors to the salon and must be displayed for all to read, should they wish. The name of the insurance company, the salon name and address, the nature of the business and the start date and renewal date will be included. Remember to renew this certificate of insurance every year.

CERTIFICATE OF EMPLOYER S LIABILITY INSURANCE (A)

(Where required by regulation 5 of the Employer's Liability (Compulsory Insurance) Regulations 1998 (the Regulations), one or more copies of this certificate must be displayed in each place of business at which the policy holder employs persons covered by the policy)

Policy No Reference No

R3/21LG52123
92L31

1. Name of policy holder — Mrs Tiffany Tsang trading as Top Tips
2. Date of commencement of insurance policy. — 31 July 2004
3. Date of expiry of insurance. — 31 July 2005

We hereby certify that subject to paragraph 2:-
1. The policy to which this certificate relates satisfies the requirements of the relevant law applicable in Great Britain, Northern Ireland, the Isle of Man, the Island of Jersey, the Island of Guernsey and the Island of Alderney (b); and
2 (a) the minimum amount of cover provided by this policy is no less than £5 million (c). Signed on behalf of EverSure plc (Authorised Insurer)
R J Stanley
CHIEF EXECUTIVE OFFICER UK

Notes
(a) Where the employer is a company to which regulation 3(2) of the Regulations applies, the certificate shall state in a prominent place, either that the policy covers the holding company and all its subsidiaries, or that the policy covers the holding company and all its subsidiaries except any specially excluded by name, or that the policy covers the holding company and only the name subsidiaries.
(b) Specify applicable law as provided for in regulation 4(5) of the Regulations.
(c) See regulation 3(1) of the Regulations and delete whichever of paragraphs 2(a) or 2(b) does not apply. Where 2(b) is applicable, specify the amount of cover provided by the relevant policy. paragraph 2(b) does not apply and is deleted.

YOUR CERTIFICATE OF EMPLOYER'S LIABILITY INSURANCE IS ATTACHED ABOVE.
THE EMPLOYER'S LIABILITY (COMPULSORY INSURANCE) REGULATIONS 1998 REQUIRE YOU TO KEEP THIS CERTIFICATE OR A COPY FOR 40 YEARS.

Please fold as shown and insert the certificate in the protective cover provided. A copy of the certificate must be displayed at all places where you employ persons covered by the policy. Extra copies of the certificate are available on request.

The insurance company requires evidence in light of a claim. They must be certain that all reasonable steps were taken to prevent the situation occurring. Were all tests carried out correctly and recorded? Were the manufacturer's instructions read, understood and followed?

Insurance companies do not always pay out on the claims that they receive if they are suspicious of negligent practices. Should this be the case, where is the money going to come from? Will the salon owner have to sell the salon? Will you have to find the money yourself?

Are you dressed for success?

First impressions are very important. People can form an opinion of you within a few minutes of meeting you. They will judge you on the way you look and the way you behave. Imagine how clients would feel if you arrived at the salon where you work looking as if you had just fallen out of bed! Do you think they would want you to do their hair if you looked like you could not take care of your own appearance?

The way you look does matter. However good your hairdressing skills may be, if you look untidy and unwashed, the image you present will give clients the wrong impression.

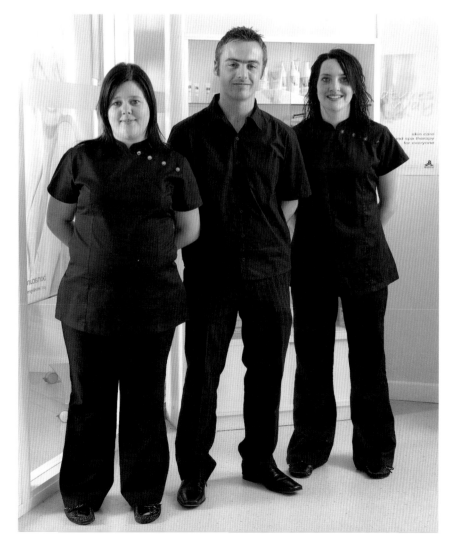

High standards of personal presentation and professional dress create a good first impression for clients

One of the most important things to remember is that the impression of any salon must be that of cleanliness, tidiness and good organisation. Your first impression when you go into a salon will help you to make your mind up whether you would want to be a client or member of staff there. If the salon appears to be clean, tidy and run efficiently you are more likely to think it is nicer than somewhere that appears to be dirty or untidy!

Personal presentation

There are many rules and regulations that will form a part of your everyday life in the salon. Equally important to the presentation of the salon is your personal presentation. Your personal presentation should be a total image – from head to foot – of acceptable safe and professional work wear.

Clothes must be neat and streamlined – so no flowing skirts, trousers or loose baggy tops. Black tends to be industry's favoured colour, although this varies from salon to salon. For safe working practices within the salon, you need to think about the most appropriate materials to wear.

Sometimes fashion shoes look great but are not always good for your feet. You will spend a lot of time on your feet when you are working in the salon and it is important to choose shoes that fit properly and meet certain health-and-safety requirements. Choose full-covered leather shoes with closed-in toes and low heels. Leather allows the feet to breathe and will help prevent unpleasant foot odour. Full-covered shoes are worn in the salon for health-and-safety reasons – they will protect your feet if you drop something sharp on to them. Sensible shoes will also stop hairs from becoming stuck in the soles of your feet!

 CHECK IT OUT

Think of reasons for the following statements about salon dress.
- Your clothes must be streamlined and not baggy.
- You must always wear full-covered shoes or boots with a low heel and sole.

Personal hygiene

Hairdressers are constantly on their feet and work in close proximity to their clients and colleagues. Your clothes must be clean and pressed on a daily basis; you must shower daily and use a suitable deodorant.

Tops must meet the waistband of your trousers or skirt – your client does not necessarily want to see your pierced navel or recent tattoo.

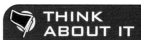

Tops must also have sleeves, short or long. When you lift your arms up to work on your clients' hair, they do not want to see your underarm hair or even smell an unwashed armpit! Smells can linger, so try to avoid spicy meals during the working week. Remember, too, that the smell of cigarette smoke can linger on your clothing or

 CHECK IT OUT

Think about other causes of bad breath. How can you avoid these?

THINK ABOUT IT

Write down the most suitable types of materials that your tops, skirts, and trousers must be made from.

Conversation topics to avoid

Conduct also falls within your personal presentation. All that you say and do is part and parcel of you as a professional person. It is pointless being correctly dressed only to follow it through with inappropriate conversation and conduct. Topics of conversation to stay away from are personal issues such as sex, drugs, religion and politics. These topics of conversation can cause friction within the salon and are best avoided. Remember that the client is your primary concern so you must demonstrate a professional business-like approach to all aspects of the client's visit.

Efficient working practices

By positioning your tools within easy reach and keeping them well organised you will make efficient use of your time and working area. Being well prepared and organised will also present a professional image to your clients. Remove waste at the end of all perming, colouring and lightening treatments and dispose of it in line with local bylaws. This will leave your working surfaces free from any risk or hazard and will present a tidy working area.

A well-organised working area will give your clients a good first impression

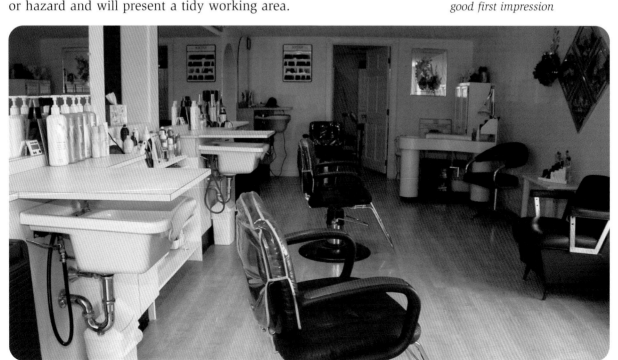

THINK ABOUT IT

Are you an extrovert who likes to show everyone how happy you are? What kind of an impression does your behaviour create? Be happy but remember that good personal conduct demonstrates to your client how professional you are. Sensible behaviour means that potential accidents are prevented, you promote a healthy and safe place to work and that the Health and Safety Act (1974) is respected.

Personal conduct

Personal conduct covers all areas of your working life, from dealing with clients and other members of staff to eating and drinking. What kind of an impression would you create if you ate in your work area?

General behaviour in the salon includes body language. If you do not agree with something, does it show in your body language? Consider whether taking drugs (prescribed legally by a doctor or obtained illegally) affects your colleagues and their clients. Always remember to check out the salon's policy for smoking and alcohol.

Finally, conduct also includes reporting staff absence and punctual timekeeping. This means that you must inform your employer of any absence and indicate your expected return date. This will give ample notice to re-organise your work schedule and allocate jobs to other members of staff.

Situation vacant

Specific duties related to health and safety should be stated in your job description and made clear to you at interview. Below is an example of a job description for you and your colleagues to discuss.

Job Description   **Post Holder Junior**
Job Title   Junior
Place of Work   Cutting Creations, Aylesbury

Candidate Specification

The successful candidate will
- Have good interpersonal skills; demonstrate a professional level of client care
- Be flexible and willing to work as a team member
- Work Saturdays and at least one late evening each week
- Take responsibility for securing models for practice and assessment purposes
- Update practical skills regularly at training sessions
- Take an active interest in all aspects of work within the salon
- Attend hairdressing seminars and professional courses in order to keep abreast of current and emerging techniques
- Demonstrate appropriate health and safety practices when working in the salon
- Complete the appropriate hairdressing qualification within the specified timeframe
- Undertake other reasonable duties as required by senior staff

Specific duties
Undertake day-to-day duties such as
- Shampoo and condition hair and scalp
- Assist with perming, relaxing, neutralising, and colouring for both European and African-Caribbean hair
- Assist with salon reception duties
- Sell retail products
- Making refreshments
- Reduce the risks to general health and safety by taking reasonable care, co-operating with requests made by senior staff and not interfering with or misusing any piece of equipment, tools or products
- Sterilise equipment
- Continuous preparation for hairdressing treatments and maintain the salon work areas
- Washing and drying towels and gowns
- Stock checking

About the salon and our staff
We are a friendly team who enjoy busy professional lives. We strive for perfection, sincerity and honesty in everything we do.

Our skills are updated on a regular basis by attending regular seminars and holding regular teach-in evenings. We look forward to working with you and wish you an enjoyable and rewarding time with us.

The candidate will enjoy
- Two weeks' paid holiday each year
- The national minimum wage
- A 40-hour working week
- 9am – 6pm (1 hour for lunch every day)

Dear Kirsty,

I have recently seen an advertisement in the local paper and I am interested in applying for the job. My hair is constantly greasy and I know that it is important to look my best when I attend interviews. I really am worried about my appearance. Can you help?

Yours sincerely,

Michelle

Kirsty says

It would be a good idea to walk into the salon and ask for their advice and guidance about controlling the excess oil that you write about. Ask about suitable products and listen to what they say about how to use the shampoo. Try using cooler water rather that hot water. Look around the salon and decide if you would like to come back for an interview or if would rather look elsewhere.

The opportunity this experience presents will stand you in good stead when dealing with prospective employers. Remember that all job interviews are different and the experience is invaluable. By taking this approach you will have obtained some sound advice about how to treat your hair and you will have made an informed decision about offering your application.

Good luck!

Kirsty

Health and safety at work

In this unit you have covered the different aspects of health and safety.

Health means being well both physically and mentally.

Safety means free from risk of danger and injury.

In order to stay well in everyday life, we need:

- clean air
- space to work and move around
- shelter, food and drink
- an ambient temperature
- and freedom of movement with no risk of harm.

Safety and comfort for you and your client

In this unit we have looked at the reasons why everyone is required to behave safely and professionally. You must take reasonable care for the health and safety of yourself and others who may be affected by what you do. You must also co-operate with your employer, salon owner or manager to ensure that health and safety procedures are followed.

You will have learnt that to work in the hairdressing industry you need to always demonstrate that you understand the health-and-safety requirements and policies in the salon. This will provide present and future employers with a professional employee who can proactively demonstrate an approved code of practice for maintaining a safe and secure working environment.

Health and safety word search

Here is a word search to help you continue with health and safety.

Find the following words in the word search below. Words can run horizontally, vertically, diagonally or backwards.

BYLAWS	PURPOSE	COOL	RISK
SAFE	H2O2	COSHH	TOP
HAZARD	WET	PPE	ROOM
FIT	HAIR	SLIPPY	POSTURE
DRUGS	HS	ENTRY	ALERT
GLOVES	TEST	EWR	PHONE
LIFT	SKIN	HANDLE	CONTAGIOUS
INFECTIOUS	INSTRUCTIONS	MANUFACTURER	

```
S  N  O  I  T  C  U  R  T  S  N  I  H  M
X  M  O  O  R  K  R  A  D  L  O  O  C  A
Y  Z  E  S  O  P  R  U  P  Z  F  I  T  N
C  C  O  N  T  A  I  G  O  U  S  N  E  U
M  S  H  2  O  2  E  T  S  A  W  F  W  F
B  A  E  C  O  S  H  H  T  O  P  E  S  A
E  F  F  V  L  X  A  F  U  D  H  C  W  C
N  E  L  I  O  Z  I  L  R  P  O  T  A  T
T  P  P  E  A  L  R  U  E  T  N  I  L  U
R  P  W  R  T  K  G  D  F  R  E  O  Y  R
Y  R  D  T  E  S  T  I  H  S  T  U  B  E
A  C  H  A  N  D  L  E  N  I  K  S  I  R
```

MEMORY JOGGER

Discuss the questions below with your colleagues. Then write down your answers.

1 What does COSHH mean?

2 What responsibilities do you have under the Electricity at Work Regulations?

3 What does RIDDOR stand for?

4 Why is it important to deal promptly with health and safety matters?

5 Why should you remain alert to the presence of hazards?

6 List three hazards within the salon.

7 Explain to a colleague the difference between a risk and a hazard.

8 Why are you asked to comply with salon requirements regarding personal presentation?

9 Why is it important to use the correct lifting technique?

10 Describe how you would deal with the following:
  a Spillages
  b Slippery surfaces
  c Obstructions to the entry and exit doors of your salon

11 Why should infectious conditions be reported to your salon manager?

12 Give an example of what might be an infectious condition.

13 How would you deal with the following situations?
  a A cut to the client's ear
  b A damaged fire extinguisher
  c Faulty electrical equipment
  d Hydrogen peroxide spillage on the floor

14 What three conditions are required for a fire to start?

15 Write down the most appropriate fire extinguisher for dealing with an electrical fire?

16 What could the possible consequences be if the incorrect fire equipment were used?

17 List three precautions that you could take to eliminate the possibility of fire.

18 Who is the person responsible for reporting health and safety matters in the salon?

19 List three safe practices for using colouring and bleaching products.

Your job role involves helping with salon reception duties. You will need to show that you can keep the reception area clean and tidy, welcome people coming into the salon, deal with their enquiries and make straightforward appointments.

The first thing to remember when working in the reception area is your own appearance! Your clothing should be neat, clean and professional looking. Choose a suitable hairstyle to reflect your salon's standards. Some make-up will also help to give you a professional look. Simple jewellery is better for working with during the day.

In this unit you will learn how to:

- maintain the reception area
- attend to clients and enquiries
- make appointments for salon services.

Your personal appearance should be as professional as your salon

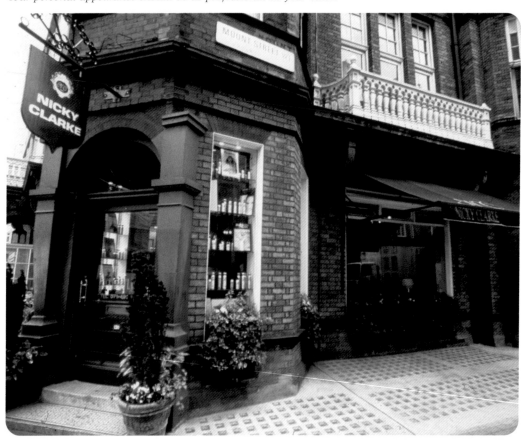

Maintain the reception area

The reception area is the first part of the salon that visitors see. You may be the first person in the salon that they come into contact with. First impressions are important. The way in which people are dealt with will affect whether they want to come back. How you handle yourself and the client will either make or break your salon's existing and future business.

CHECK IT OUT

What is your salon's policy for client care at reception?

The reception area – is it clean and tidy?

Is your salon reception area clean, tidy and welcoming? Put yourself in the place of a client and look at your reception critically. Would you feel as if you were in a professional salon? Not all salons have a separate reception area, but even so the area in which the client is welcomed must be professionally presented. It is your duty to make sure that the reception area is clean and tidy at all times.

THINK ABOUT IT

Think about the limits of your own authority when working in reception. Are there certain things that you can and cannot do when dealing with people and their enquiries and making appointments?

Who do you refer reception problems to?

The reception area is the 'shop window' of the salon – it needs to give clients a good impression

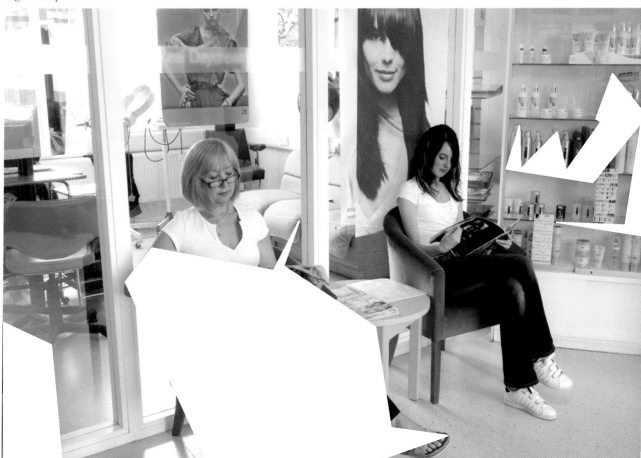

Retail products

Your salon may sell a range of retail products. It is your job to display these neatly and to make sure that the display is kept fully stocked and dust free. This will encourage clients to look at the products and will also help them to decide whether they want to pick up the product.

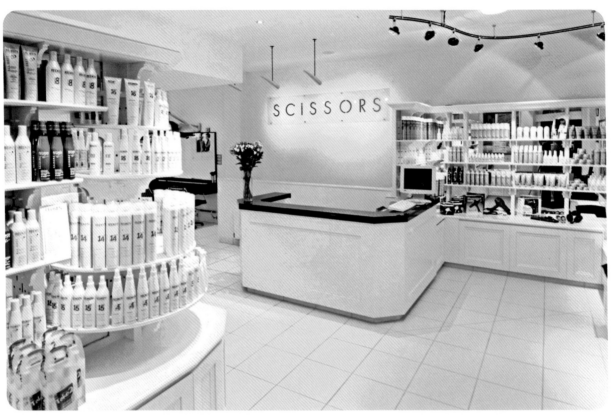

Retail product displays should look good so clients are tempted to buy!

 CHAT ROOM

Did you know that women spend more on retail products than men?

This type of work is best done when the salon is quiet. It may be first thing in the morning or there may be quiet times during the day when you could dust and rearrange the products on display.

Remember that all staff must be fully aware of products stocked by the salon and how to use them.

Security of stock

It is vital to keep the salon's stock secure. Small items can be removed easily without anyone noticing. The thief may be a visitor to the salon or even a member of staff. Stock should be regularly checked against actual sales to show whether anything is missing.

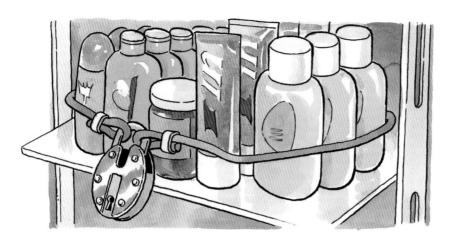

Make it difficult for thieves to take your salon's stock

CHAT ROOM

Where products are on display, think about using empty boxes or bottles. This will help to prevent theft. If stock losses can be kept to a minimum, this will directly affect your salon's final profit.

Low levels of stock

You will need a variety of resources such as stationery to help you to do your job. Take a regular stock check of pencils, erasers, pencil sharpeners, rulers, appointment pages/books, products and message pads. Check also that you have enough change in the till!

THINK ABOUT IT

Make a simple list of the most popular salon retail products and list the cost of each product. You may find this information useful when dealing with enquiries.

CHECK IT OUT

Who should you report low levels of stationery and products to in your salon?

WELLA HAIR PRODUCTS	
Wella Lifetex Shampoo	£3.50
Wella Lifetex Mousse Conditioners	£3.80
Wella Lifetex Intensive Conditioners	£3.60
Wella High Hair Product Samples	99p each or 3 for £2.50
Wella Hair Mascara	£2.50

A retail products list

Promptly reporting stock shortages can make the difference between offering a professional service and making an appointment, closing a sale, or irritating the client by making him or her wait.

Faulty products

Sometimes accidents happen and stock may become damaged. Remove all faulty products from the reception area as soon as you can and report them to the person who controls the stock. Look for faulty stock as you prepare it for sale, for example damaged or loose packaging, cracks or splits in bottles, leaks, and so on.

Removing faulty products is essential to the smooth running of the reception area and can mean the difference between a client buying a product or not. Many salons operate a commission on all retail products sold, so it pays to be alert when dealing with stock.

Looking after your clients

Clients like to be looked after. Remember to offer them a drink and something to read. Your salon may have a client care policy of offering alcoholic and non-alcoholic drinks. This is sometimes free to the client as part of the salon's hospitality policy.

It is good practice to offer refreshments when clients are waiting for the stylist to attend to them. It gives the client a feeling that something is happening.

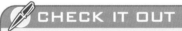
CHECK IT OUT

In your salon:

1. Do you know where the cups and saucers are kept?

2. Where would you find clean glasses?

3. Children may want a soft drink. Do you have plastic glasses?

4. Where do you get more stock of coffee, tea, sugar and milk?

Attend to clients and enquiries

Imagine that you have walked into a salon for the first time and you want to find out how much a haircut is? How would you feel to be a client? The salon reception area is often a busy place, so when carrying out reception duties you will need to behave professionally at all times.

Welcoming people is what your job is all about. Make them feel special and let them see that you are pleased to see them.

A positive and polite manner

Communication is a vital part of reception work. It is important to the success of the business.

There are two types of communication:

- Verbal communication uses the spoken word, either face to face or over the telephone.
- Non-verbal communication does not use the spoken word, for example when you write down a message or an appointment for a client. It can also mean the body language that you use such as nodding, smiling, frowning, listening and sign language.

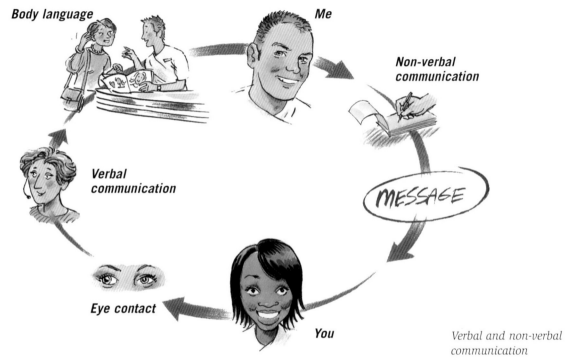

Verbal and non-verbal communication

Communication needs to be effective and clear to everyone involved. When a client makes an appointment, you will need to repeat the information back to him or her to make sure that both you and the client understand the same thing.

Written messages must be clear. It is often a good idea to take the message to the person concerned for his or her immediate attention.

Smile when dealing with people making enquiries, be attentive and help them in a positive and polite manner. This will help the person to decide if he or she wants to return to your salon. Always show positive body language – clients may pick up on negative body language.

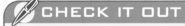 CHECK IT OUT

Discuss with a colleague positive and negative body language when dealing with clients.

Identifying the purpose of the enquiry

Not all visitors coming into the salon will want to make an appointment. They may have come to deliver an order or to read the water meter. Whatever the nature of the enquiry, find out what it is as soon as possible. If you are busy, acknowledge the person and indicate that you will be with him or her shortly.

The enquiry could come from a telephone call. For example, it might be a technical rep who is new to the area needing directions to your salon. Locate a map of the local area showing where the salon is and keep it handy just in case you need to help someone find their way.

Should you need another member of staff to help you, tell the visitor that you will not be long and seek further assistance promptly.

An efficient, friendly manner will give a good first impression of how the salon deals with visitors.

Confirming appointments

The salon's business is driven by those who operate the appointments system. It may be that your salon has a manual appointments system – appointments are written in pencil in an appointments book.

Some salons have a computer-based appointments system whereby you can make clients' appointments directly on to the screen.

As soon as the client comes into the salon, ask how you can help and identify the client's appointment as efficiently as you can. Suggest to your client that he or she might like to take a seat while you inform the stylist of the client's arrival. This is also a good opportunity to practise your client-care policy by offering refreshments and magazines.

Recording messages

The importance of passing on messages to the right people at the right time often requires diplomacy and tact. You must be able to read the situation in the salon before rushing in to pass on a message. You will need to learn how and when to ask questions and to say things that suit the purpose of the call.

Below are some typical situations that you may have to deal with.

The senior stylist is busy with a client. Her mum rings with an important message. It is often best to check if the stylist is able to come to the telephone to take the call and, if not, write down the message.

When writing down a message, use your salon's message pad. Listen carefully to the caller before writing down the message. Read it back to confirm accuracy. Take the message to the stylist or the person concerned and pass any reply back to the caller. Give all information clearly and accurately and make sure all confidential information is given only to authorised people.

A caller may be complaining about a service he or she has received and might ask to speak to the manager. In situations such as this, you will need to be calm, responsible and tactful. Using the salon message pad, write down as much information from the client as you can. Show the client that you are listening by confirming the details. Keep your tone of voice objective without taking sides. Ask the client politely to hold on, then take the message to a senior member of staff and await instructions.

It may be that the manager is too busy to speak or respond to the client and the manager may need to phone back. You may be asked to tell the client this. Speak clearly to avoid any confusion.

MESSAGE

FOR	Deepak
FROM	Mrs Alessi
TEL. NO.	0208 321 145

TELEPHONED ✓   PLEASE RING ✓

CALLED TO SEE YOU ☐   WILL CALL AGAIN ☐

WANTS TO SEE YOU ☐   URGENT ☐

MESSAGE: Needs to speak to you asap – you can call her on the tel. no. above up to 5.30pm

DATE: 10.05.02   TIME: 9.03am

RECEIVED BY: Amber

Use the salon's message pad to take down messages

CHECK IT OUT

1 What is your salon's policy for taking and recording messages?

2 Discuss with a colleague what to do in each of the following situations:
   a A client rings for a treatment list and tariff.
   b The wholesaler rings to confirm the salon's order.
   c A future bride is enquiring about the cost of three hair-up styles?

Confidential information

What is confidential information?

In the salon, this will include:

- the contents of client records
- client and staff personal details such as name, address and telephone number
- financial matters relating to the business.

Sometimes personal conversations with colleagues may be confidential.

Confidential information should only be given to authorised people.

Data Protection Act (1998)

Under this Act, you must not pass on any personal information to another person without the permission of the person involved. Your salon may obtain, hold and use personal data which is relevant for its own use.

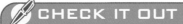
CHECK IT OUT

1 Find out what your salon's procedures are for maintaining confidentiality.

2 What might the consequence be if you break the salon's confidentiality policy.

Make appointments for salon services

THINK ABOUT IT

Write down the differences between using an appointment book and a computer when making clients' appointments.

People contact the salon in a variety of ways. It could be that they telephone, visit the salon, or a friend may make an appointment on their behalf, or they may send an email or text message to enquire about an appointment. You will need to know about the services that the salon offers together with the products and available times that you can offer an appointment.

Information such as each stylist's lunch hour, start and finish times, day off and late night worked is all part of how your salon operates and it will help you to know this when making appointments.

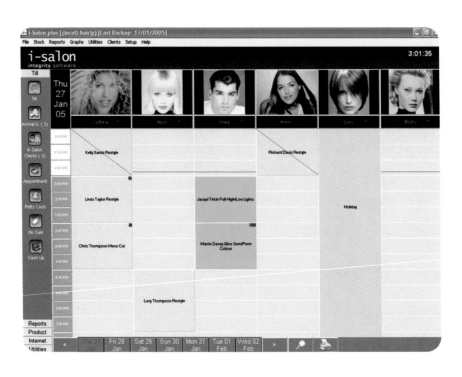

Page from an electronic appointments book

Services such as cuts, blow-dries, sets, conditioning treatments and hair-up styles are non-chemical treatments. Colours, perms, relaxers, bleach, highlights and lowlights are chemical treatments.

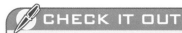

CHECK IT OUT

Find out the cost of non-chemical and chemical treatments offered by your salon. Clients may ask you for this information when they make an appointment.

The salon will set aside a specific amount of time for each service. For example, it may take a few hours to complete a chemical service, while a cut or set may take less than an hour. You must make sure that you leave enough time for each service to be finished professionally.

CHECK IT OUT

1 Confirm with the stylist how long to leave for each service.

2 What is your salon's procedure for making and recording appointments?

When making an appointment always make sure that you deal with the request politely and promptly.

Identifying the client's requirements

Your client's request may take a few minutes to deal with and may cover a range of services offered by the salon. The client may be making an appointment for several people and this will need your patience and knowledge of how the salon operates.

Look at the appointment page and find out who is free and who will be able to offer each of these services. If you are not sure how to deal with a particular appointment request, then you should ask a senior member of staff for assistance.

Confirming appointment details

Your client's name, telephone number, service requested, date, time and member of staff booked for the service must always be discussed and confirmed with the client when he or she makes an appointment.

Repeat the information for the appointment to the client and ask if it is acceptable. If the client is in the salon, ask whether he or she would like an appointment card with the details written down.

On the appointment page or computer screen, make sure that all of the information is recorded accurately, in the right place, at the right time and that you have left sufficient time to complete the service.

If using a manual appointment system, make sure that your writing is neat and easy to read. Use a pencil to make appointments and if need be, rub out any mistakes or cancellations. This helps to make good use of the available space on the page and keeps it clear and easy to follow.

Telephone appointments

Many appointments are made by phone. When answering the phone, smile – the client can hear the difference in your tone of voice! Listen carefully to what the client is saying and make each appointment as promptly as you can.

Using the phone properly and efficiently is important to the smooth running of the salon business. It can be the first point of contact between you and the client. On answering the phone, remember to tell the caller the name of the salon and who you are, for example 'Good morning, Head Start, Laura speaking, how can I help you?'. As soon as the caller tells you his or her name, start to use it. It gives the caller a feeling of confidence that you have listened to basic information and that you have begun to develop a professional relationship.

Always answer the phone professionally

If you need to discuss appointment details with a colleague, it is a good idea not to leave the client holding on listening to salon

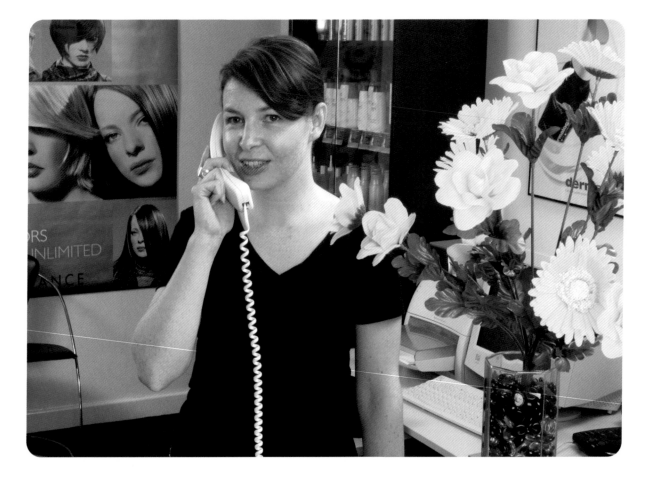

background noise. Most phones have a mute button which will allow you to talk to your colleague without the caller hearing. Don't forget to press the mute button again when you return to speak to the client, otherwise he or she will not hear you! Repeat the information back to the client and check that he or she is happy with the appointment time, date and stylist.

If you are making an appointment for a client who would like a permanent colour which touches the skin, you must remember to offer a skin test. Skin tests are recommended by the manufacturer and should be carried out 24–48 hours before the permanent colour application.

Complete the appointment booking by saying 'Thank you' and 'We look forward to seeing you' followed by 'Goodbye' or 'See you soon'.

 CHECK IT OUT

With a colleague, practise making appointments for the following clients:
- Mrs Hodgart would like a blow dry. She has long hair.
- Mrs Spyrou would like a perm and cut.
- Mr Stevenson would like a dry cut.
- Miss Iqbal would like highlights on medium-length hair.
- Mr Schneider would like a beard trim.

 MEMORY JOGGER

Discuss the questions below with your colleagues. Then write down your answers.

1 List the information needed when making an appointment.

2 When the phone rings, how soon should you answer it?

3 When answering the phone, what should you say?

4 List your salon's rules of confidentiality.

5 What may happen if you break the salon's rules of confidentiality?

6 How should your client's personal information be treated?

7 What are the different types of communication?

8 Give an example of each type of communication.

9 Who should you refer difficult clients to?

10 Why should you use a pencil when making an appointment?

11 Give two reasons why appointments need to be made correctly.

12 What types of payment methods does your salon accept?

13 Why does the reception area need to be clean and tidy?

Salon reception duties word search

Find the following words in the word search below.
Words can run horizontally or vertically.

TARIFF	INFORMATION	COMPUTER
ENQUIRIES	COMMUNICATION	PROFESSIONAL
COFFEE	LOOK SMART ALWAYS	TABLE
OFFER	FLOWERS	MAGAZINE RACK
TELEPHONE	MAT	SUGAR
TEA	COST	PRICES
SALON	TIME	CLIENT
EMAIL	CASH	APPOINTMENT
PENCIL	SEND	ANGRY

```
X  M  A  G  A  Z  I  N  E  R  A  C  K  L  J  A  C
M  S  C  O  M  M  U  N  I  C  A  T  I  O  N  J  S
P  C  O  S  T  C  U  D  O  R  P  E  N  C  I  L  D
R  W  N  F  L  O  W  E  R  S  P  M  F  S  Y  K  F
O  F  F  E  R  G  H  S  A  L  O  N  O  U  T  H  G
F  Y  C  O  M  P  U  T  E  R  I  P  R  G  F  X  W
E  J  K  L  M  A  C  L  I  E  N  T  M  A  T  Q  T
S  T  E  L  E  P  H  O  N  E  T  E  A  R  A  P  A
S  E  N  S  S  E  N  D  S  T  M  R  T  N  R  O  B
I  M  T  X  U  R  P  R  I  C  E  S  I  L  I  M  L
O  A  I  A  A  T  I  M  E  U  N  C  O  F  F  E  E
N  I  A  N  G  R  Y  R  H  C  T  V  N  T  F  I  C
A  L  L  C  E  N  Q  U  I  R  I  E  S  C  A  S  H
L  O  O  K  S  M  A  R  T  A  L  W  A  Y  S  C  P
```

A happy salon is a pleasant place to work in and to visit. Good working relationships with both clients and colleagues are essential to the smooth running of the salon. This unit will help you to develop effective working relationships.

A client's trust and goodwill must be earned. Showing you can do your own job well will give clients confidence in your ability. If you upset a client or behave in an unprofessional way, the client may not come back to the salon. On the other hand, if the client is happy with your work, he or she is likely to return.

You are very much a part of a team as you work in the salon. This unit will help you to work as a support to all around you. In this way, you can aim to be an effective team member.

This unit will also give you the chance to find out the best ways to develop your skills within your job role. You will then be ready to move on in your chosen career.

In this unit you will learn how to:

- develop effective working relationships with clients
- develop effective working relationships with colleagues
- develop yourself within your job role.

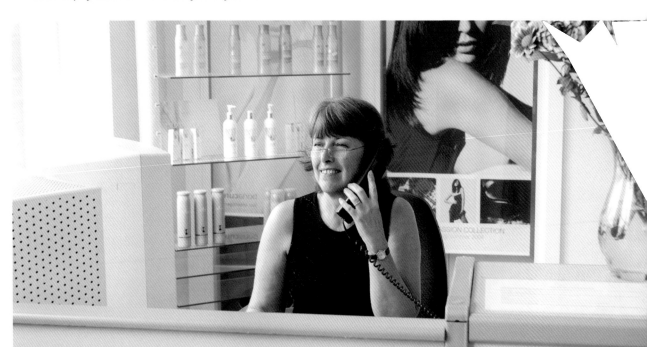

Develop effective working relationships with clients

Communicating with clients

Clients are the most important part of your work. You will need to treat them with respect. In turn, this should encourage their goodwill and help them to trust you. Always remember to maintain client confidentiality.

Communicate clearly with your clients. A calm, confident and polite manner is important. Speak in a friendly way to all visitors to the salon and, of course, to your own staff team.

When speaking to clients, try to attract and keep eye contact. Think about how to listen and focus on what the client is saying. Positive body language is essential. Use your eyes to express yourself positively and remember to smile – you will put the client at ease if you appear welcoming. Sometimes clients may be shy and timid and it can take skill to encourage them to talk to you.

> **THINK ABOUT IT**
>
> How would you feel if you were trying to speak to someone and the person appeared bored or did not bother to look at you?

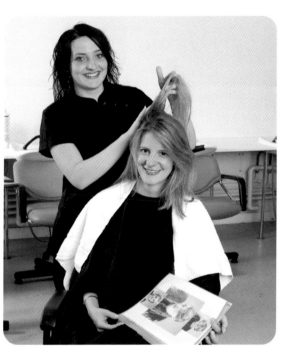

Listen carefully to what the client is saying

Handling clients' personal items

Often clients will trust you to take care of their belongings. Look in your reception area to see if there is a sign which makes it clear that the salon does not take responsibility for personal belongings. Whatever your salon policy for clients' belongings, it must be communicated clearly to them.

Nevertheless, you should handle clients' belongings with reasonable care. There may be coat hooks or even a wardrobe where you can hang clients' clothing. Any client would expect you to handle personal items with respect and return them at the end of the visit.

Dealing with client concerns

There are many mirrors in the salon and you will need to learn to use them for different purposes. Think about using the mirror to hold a conversation, or to look at the hairstyle as it is developing. You can also use the mirror to check for signs of unhappiness, or if the client is confused or angry.

To be an effective team member, you must make sure that the client's comfort and needs are dealt with confidentially and professionally.

It may be that the client's concern is within your responsibilities, and you can deal with it in a professional way. Should you ever need to discuss a client's concern, you should know who to report the matter to. The salon manager is usually the person to report difficult situations to. Always work within your salon's client-care policy and deal with the concern promptly and efficiently. This will encourage the client's trust and goodwill.

 CHAT ROOM

If clients have a complaint, remember to let them know how it is being dealt with. No one likes to be kept waiting, so deal with queries and concerns promptly!

 CHECK IT OUT

How would you recognise signs that your client is angry or confused?

Your appearance and behaviour

Your standard of behaviour must be professional at all times. The way staff behave, either when dealing with clients or between clients, will be noticed by everyone in the salon.

Remember, too, the importance of a professional image. Wearing the appropriate salon uniform, make-up and a suitable professional hairstyle that reflects your salon's standards will show clients that you have taken care of yourself, and this will help you to build a professional relationship with them.

Client comfort

Look after your clients. Offer them a drink, magazines and perhaps discuss alternative treatments. Always offer them the same level of professionalism on each and every visit. Ask simple questions to make sure they are comfortable and to let them know that you have thought about their comfort and care.

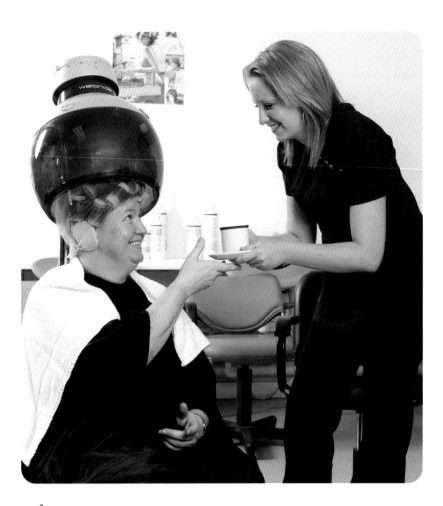

The client's comfort is very important

 CHAT ROOM

It is the extra mile that you go with clients that will encourage them to come back to your salon!

 CHECK IT OUT

Think of three reasons why you should look after the client's comfort.

Develop effective working relationships with colleagues

Teamwork is vital to the smooth running of the salon. You will need to be sure that your staff team is happy with how you are carrying out your job role.

Being courteous

A happy salon environment makes a good impression on clients. Staff working well together – helping each other in a team – will help to create a good atmosphere. As well as being friendly and respectful to clients, you must also be friendly and respectful to colleagues.

CHAT ROOM

Smile – you will look great and you will feel great!

Asking for and giving help

When asking colleagues for help and information, you should be polite. Sometimes it is not what you ask for, but the way in which you ask for it. If a colleague asks for your help, always give it willingly.

CHECK IT OUT

With a colleague, practise asking for an early lunch hour, using both positive and negative types of communication.

What types of response did you get?

Making efficient use of your time

Stylists and managers expect to receive a speedy and efficient service from their staff, which is you! You will need to use your time efficiently which in turn will help the salon to run smoothly.

In a salon, time is money. It is essential that your time and your colleagues' time is used effectively. In practice, this means making sure everything is prepared ready for the stylist to move on to the next client.

CHECK IT OUT

Alan, a junior stylist at Cool Cutz, finishes work at 6 pm. He has a 10-minute walk home. There are several activities he needs to do this evening and he wants to have finished everything by 11.30 pm.

- Alan has a chapter of his hairdressing book to read tonight – 50 minutes.
- He needs to revise for a major written paper – 40 minutes.
- There is a project, which his tutor is reminding him about – 35 minutes.
- He wants to spend time emailing his girlfriend – 15 minutes.
- His favourite program is on TV at 8.30 pm – 90 minutes.
- He also wants to spend an hour jogging round the park.

With a colleague, work out how Alan can make effective use of his time. Remember to leave time for him to have a quick evening meal!

Assisting colleagues

Your job includes passing up tools and equipment such as rollers, pins, perm papers and perm rods to the stylist. You should pass these in such a way that enables the stylist to progress more quickly with the treatment. This will help the stylist to make efficient use of his or her time.

Making coffee for clients, cleaning the backwash basins, sweeping the floor, maintaining record cards, carrying out skin tests, flushing the hot water through first thing in the morning, and replacing the barbicide are all part of your responsibilities.

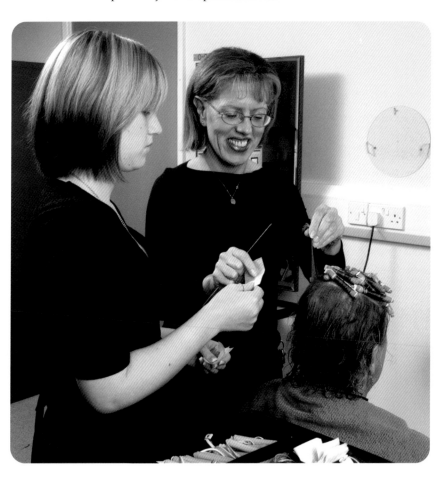

You will need to assist the stylist to carry out treatments

 CHAT ROOM

Your efficiency at work will help the salon to run smoothly, and will benefit all staff. The clients will be happy and you may be able to earn more commission!

You can also assist colleagues by ensuring that the reception area is clean and tidy, and all retail shelves are neatly displayed and fully stocked. Keep the salon tidy by clearing away used towels, used cups and saucers, and tinting bowls, which need to be rinsed out.

Some of the hands-on hair treatments that you will be asked to do will involve shampooing, colour removal, neutralising, conditioning treatments, removing rollers, removing perm rods and preparing the hair for further treatments such as sectioning for the stylist to apply the colour.

 CHAT ROOM

If the client is worried about lots of hair in the comb or brush, reassure him or her that it is perfectly normal. You can lose up to 100 hairs each day.

If you run out of any product or resource that is needed to provide a professional service, you must report it straightaway to the relevant person.

Below is a simple acronym that will help you to remember what teamwork is all about:

Together
Everyone
Achieves
More

 CHECK IT OUT

❶ What teams are you part of? How do you feel when people do not play their part?

❷ Discuss with a colleague how you would fit into an existing team of staff.

Develop yourself within your job role

You are an important member of staff who is central to the success of all treatments that take place within the salon. Your role is to help your team as much as you can, all day and everyday. Your colleagues are relying on you to carry out your job in a professional way. Do not let them or your clients down by failing to turn up at work.

All staff need to be motivated and aim to offer their clients a professional service. Good working relationships are important to the smooth running of the salon and all staff must be happy to take part in whatever job needs doing.

Seeking agreement

Sometimes you may need to check a procedure with a senior manager. Always treat a manager with the respect his or her position deserves. Managers have worked hard to achieve their job role and are in a position to assist you if you show them that you are serious about your career.

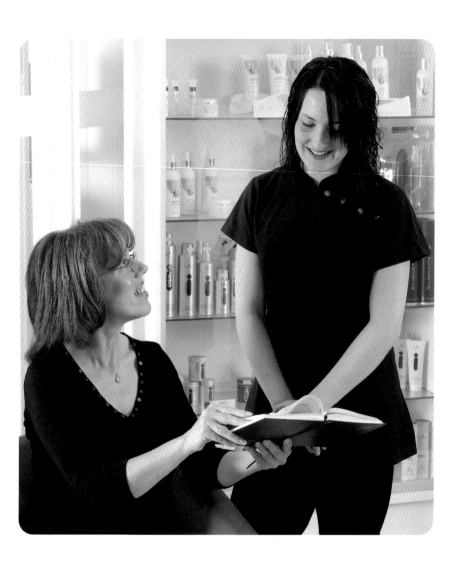

If you need time off, ask the salon manager's permission

If you need time off, make sure that you have a genuine reason and ask politely for the manager's agreement.

 CHECK IT OUT

With a colleague, write a list of genuine reasons for taking time off from work.

Working within your responsibilities

If you are asked to do a task but are unsure how to do it, or the instructions you have are unclear, check with the relevant person how to proceed.

Always work within the limits of your job role. The consequences could be serious if you were to carry out a treatment that you had not been trained to do.

Use equipment for the purpose intended and check that it is safe to use. If you are in doubt, ask a senior member of staff.

Keeping up professional standards

Your behaviour and personal appearance, including personal hygiene, must be of a high standard at all times. Attendance and punctuality are very important too.

 CHECK IT OUT

Good staff are hard to find. List the qualities of a good member of staff.

Your professional development

How you develop yourself in your job role is important to your own professional development and to the success of the salon.

By identifying the most appropriate person in the salon who can provide professional staff training and working with that person, you will be able to develop your own personal training plan for success.

An experienced stylist instructing a junior stylist on how to use a hood steamer

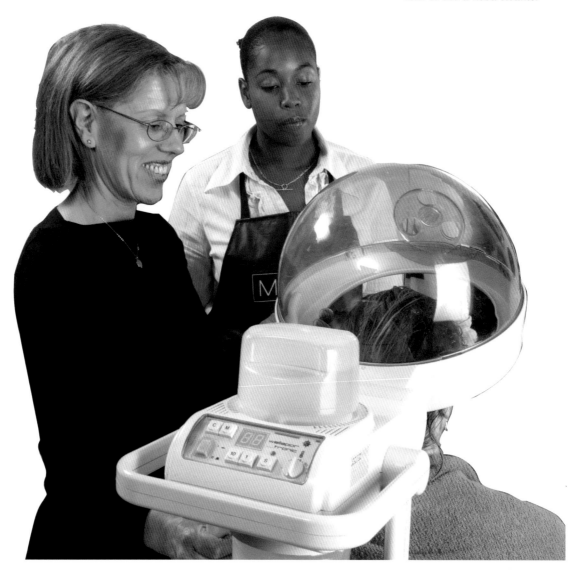

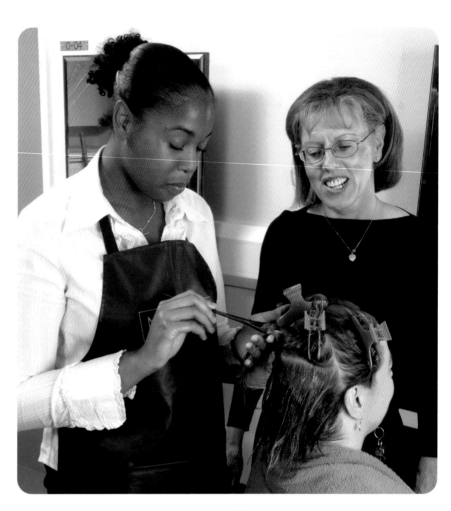

A junior stylist being trained to apply a conditioning treatment

Using the existing framework of qualifications as a guide, make your plan. When you have developed your own professional record, keep it up to date. Many of your senior colleagues will be able to help with this as it is also part of their job to keep themselves up to date.

Discuss your personal training plan with your supervisor and plan how you are going to achieve areas for further development. Remember to include a review date where you can sit down together to review your progress.

 CHECK IT OUT

Make an action plan. Start by listing the types of things you want to improve, for example shampooing or neutralising. Think about the future and what you want to achieve.

Carrying out your action plan will help you to:

- develop your strengths
- focus on areas for further development
- promote good working relationships within the salon
- become more effective at your job in the salon.

It is a good idea to keep a daily record of the type of work you do so that you and your manager can reflect on what you are doing. Remember to ask colleagues for feedback to help you improve your performance. It is best to have a weekly review so that your memory is clear and a positive discussion can take place.

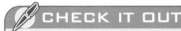

CHECK IT OUT

How can you identify your own strengths and areas for further development?

Understanding instructions

You may find the instructions you have been given to carry out a task are not clear. If so, discuss the appropriate course of action with a senior member of staff. This will make sure that you know exactly what you have to do. The job will then be carried out correctly, you will avoid misusing a product, client comfort and satisfaction will be maintained and this will help to promote a professional image.

Learning opportunities

Everyone learns differently. You may learn best by watching the stylist at work, or by listening to instructions either before or while you are doing a task.

Take advantage of all the skills that are being demonstrated everyday by senior staff. You can also learn when assisting stylists. Look at how they stand or hold their hands when carrying out a treatment. Look at the client's hair before, during and after the service so that you can see how the style develops.

There are many opportunities to learn and develop your professional skills. Try visiting some of the shows and exhibitions that are held every year to see top stylists demonstrate hair-up styles, cuts, colours and many more interesting and exciting aspects of the hairdressing industry.

Watch some of the many TV channels that show hairdressing salons and the many and varied types of work that they are involved in. Keep up to date with techniques and products by reading the weekly *Hairdressers Journal*.

Look at pop stars, movie stars, and so on, to find out what are the latest fashions. Hairdressing is all about fashion and you must be up to date. Attend each and every staff training session and take part in the salon's training and development plan. Watch technical services and ask questions about what you see and why it is happening that way.

Setting self-development targets and reviewing progress

Many salons will expect you to achieve S/NVQ Level 1 within one year. It is possible to achieve this qualification within that time, which would then mean you could be considered for an S/NVQ Level 2 training programme.

Keep up to date with the latest styles, techniques and products

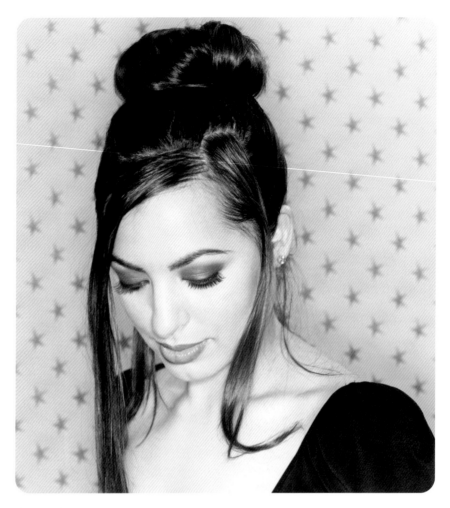

You and your salon should set realistic targets in which to achieve units of work. You must take personal responsibility for your own targets and understand the importance of meeting them. The salon owner may be unhappy if you fail to do so!

A calendar showing progression and achievement would be a useful piece of evidence to develop. This should show clearly what you need to do and by what date. It could also set out the salon's commitment to you as a staff member in terms of training. Review your progress regularly with your manager and use this to develop any further action that may be needed.

Meeting your self-development targets should lead to increased job satisfaction, the opportunity to progress to other tasks within hairdressing and to attract a higher financial reward.

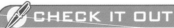 **CHECK IT OUT**

With two colleagues, draw up an action plan/calendar of progression leading to achievement.

Discuss the results with your manager.

Procedures

Your job description and contract of employment

When you attend an interview, the job description – a list of the specific and general duties you will be expected to do – should be discussed. Once you start work at the salon, a copy of the job description will be placed in your records. Make sure you read it carefully and do what it says.

You should be given a contract of employment within three months of starting your job.

Salon meetings

Most salons hold regular meetings and this is the time to discuss general issues that may concern you. Anything of a private nature must be kept confidential such as staff details, client details, salon details and any disciplinary proceedings. Remember, if you breach the salon's policy for confidentiality, you could be disciplined.

JOB DESCRIPTION – JUNIOR

Job title: Junior
Place of work: Cutting Creations, Banbury

Candidate specification
About the candidate
The candidate should:
- have good interpersonal skills and demonstrate a professional level of client care
- have the flexibility and willingness to work as a team member
- be able to work on Saturday and at least one late evening each week
- take responsibility for securing models for practise and assessment purposes
- update practical skills regularly at training sessions
- take an active interest in all aspects of work within the salon
- attend hairdressing seminars and professional courses in order to keep up to date with current and emerging techniques
- complete the appropriate hairdressing qualification within the specified time frame
- undertake other reasonable duties, from time to time, as required by senior staff.

Specific duties
Undertake day-to-day duties such as:
- shampoo and condition hair and scalp
- assist with perming, relaxing, neutralising and colouring for both European and African-Caribbean hair
- assist with salon reception duties
- sell retail products
- make refreshments
- reduce the risks to general health and safety
- sterilise equipment
- prepare hairdressing treatments and maintain the salon work areas (continuous)
- wash and dry towels and gowns
- check stock.

About the salon and our staff
We are a friendly team who enjoy busy professional lives. We strive for perfection, sincerity and honesty in everything we do. Our skills are updated regularly by attending seminars and holding teach-in evenings. We look forward to working with you and wish you an enjoyable and rewarding time with us.

The candidate will enjoy:
- two weeks paid holiday each year
- a 37-hour working week
- the national minimum wage
- 9 am starts and one hour for lunch every day.

Job description

The salon's appeals and grievance procedure

The salon will have copies of its appeals and grievance procedure, which all members of staff should have access to. If you have a grievance, deal with the problem sensibly, calmly, professionally and seek independent advice on how to deal with the situation.

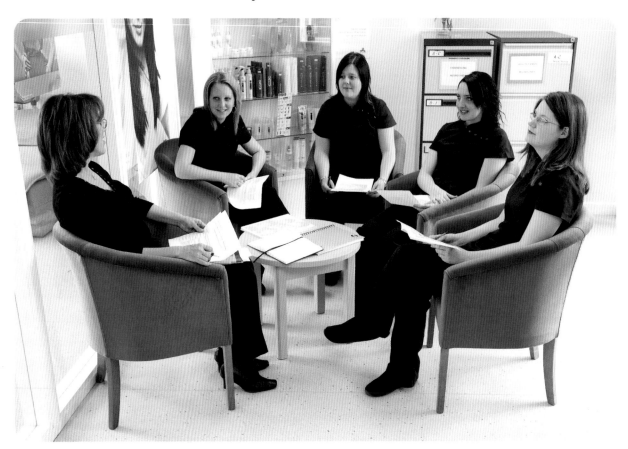

Most salons hold team meetings to discuss general issues

Working relationships word search

Find the following words in the word search opposite. Words can run horizontally, vertically, diagonally or backwards.

BEHAVIOUR	SALON	ACHIEVES
MANNER	ALL	TOGETHER
PRODUCTS	HELP	EVERY
MILE	SHAMPOO	VERBAL
CUTS	RINSE	TEAMWORK
COLOUR	VISUAL	TENDER
REMOVAL	NEUTRALISING	SALE
RECORDS	GOWNED	HAPPY
CLIENT CARE	PAID	LOVING
SUPPORT	HARMONY	CARE
PROFESSIONAL	DELIVERY	COMMUNICATION
ONE	EXIT	RECEPTION
MOTIVATIONAL	TOOLS	MORE

```
R S K D E L I V E R Y S W E V E O
H D C R X J S C A C H I E V E S T
C R A K I G O W N E D O N E R N R
N O P C T X T O G E T H E R B I O
E C L C L I E N T C A R E Y A R P
U E E O G P A I D Y J A C L L U P
T R H M A S M M O R E C O X I Y U
R N S M R Y W L C E L U N I C M S
A O T U U M O T I V A T I O N A L
L I C N O P R O F E S S I O N A L
I T U I L U K R E M O V A L T L L
S P D C O C N O L A S Y X O E A A
I E O A C H I E V E P L C V N U S
N C R T X S H A M P O O A I D S L
G E P I P O S M A N N E R N E I O
P R U O I V A H E B N S E G R V O
Q S Y N O M R A H A W M H C M B T
```

⚡ MEMORY JOGGER

Discuss the questions below with your colleagues. Then write down your answers.

1 Discuss how each of the following methods of communication can be used professionally within the salon:
   a written
   b verbal
   c non-verbal.

2 List the reasons for making sure client comfort is maintained.

3 Identify ways in which you could maintain client comfort.

4 What may happen if you break the salon rules of confidentiality?

5 Why should you work positively within a team?

6 What might happen if you ignore the manufacturer's or stylist's instructions?

7 Explain the benefits of continued professional development.

8 Why should you respond positively to reviews from staff?

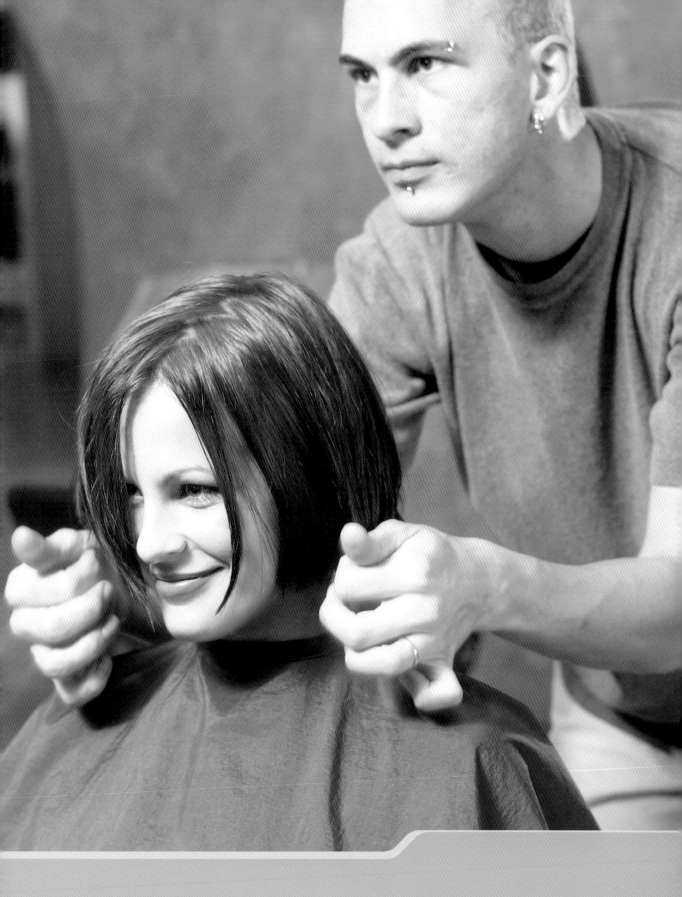

PRACTICAL SKILLS

When working in the salon, you will be expected to follow health, safety and hygiene procedures. You will need to show that you have met the standards for preparation and maintaining hairdressing work areas.

Everything you have learned so far about health and safety and COSHH needs to be brought together in this unit. (To remind yourself of health and safety in the salon, see Unit G1 Ensure your own actions reduce risks to health and safety.) Your assessor will observe your performance which must include preparation for different hairdressing treatments, that is ladies' services and/or barbering.

In this unit you will learn how to:

■ prepare for hairdressing services
■ maintain the work area for hairdressing services.

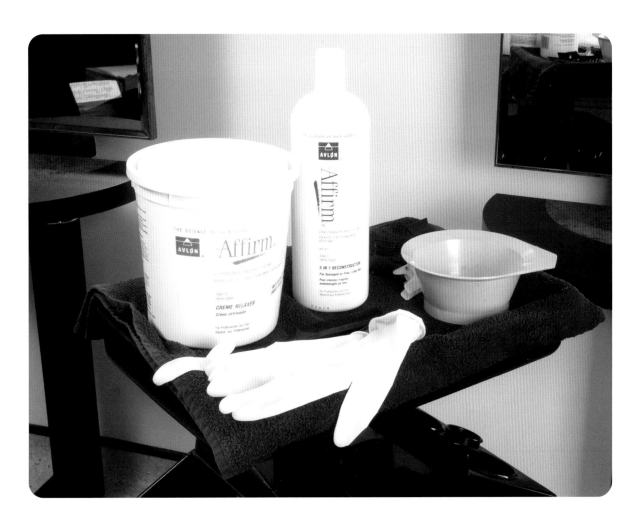

Prepare for hairdressing treatments

Preparing hairdressing tools and materials takes place everyday within many salons, both in colleges and in training centres. Instructions must be followed and your own salon policy adhered to. Your stylist or senior manager will instruct you about what is needed on a daily basis. As you work with your team, you will soon get to know how each staff member works and what he or she requires.

Setting up materials, tools and equipment

Think about the type of work that has been booked in for the day. There may be several perms, some colours, a relaxer and a conditioning treatment. You will need to prepare for each treatment separately.

For example, the stylist will need a perm tray for each perm which should include:

- different sized rods
- end papers for perming
- tension strips
- barrier cream
- the appropriate perming lotion and neutraliser.

Similarly, you will need to set up a tray for colouring treatments.

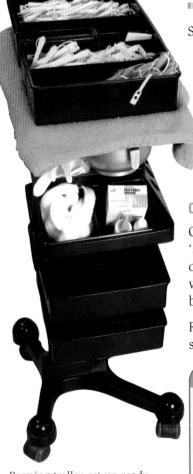

Perming trolley set up ready for the stylist

> ### CHECK IT OUT
>
> Find out:
> - what to put on a perm tray
> - how to set up for a colour
> - how to set up for a conditioning treatment
> - where the record cards are kept in your salon.

Observation

Observation plays a major part in many hairdressing salons. Staff can 'speak' to each other using eye contact rather than language. Look out for signs and learn to identify your team's body language. This will help you anticipate the needs of other people, which in turn will benefit both clients and colleagues.

Remember to observe, not stare! Make sure that when you watch someone it is for a professional purpose.

> ### CHECK IT OUT
>
> Look for signs that your team may need something such as a comb or a pair of clippers.
>
> Watch what each staff member uses – he or she may have a favourite comb or brush. Does this need to be sterilised before the next client?

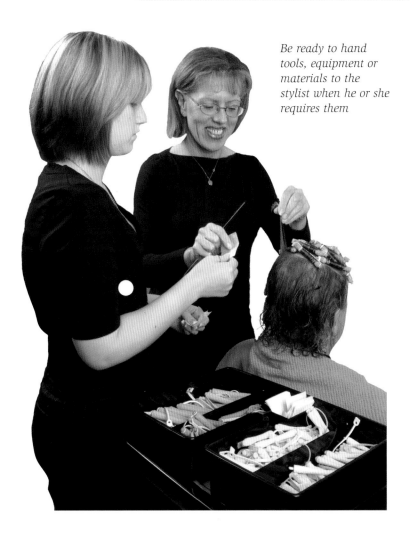

Be ready to hand tools, equipment or materials to the stylist when he or she requires them

Preparing in time for the treatment

Timing in the salon is everything – sometimes things can happen too soon or not soon enough. Think about the products you may need at the end of a treatment. It could be serum, hairspray, wax, or a mixture of different products. Be on the look out for opportunities to assist your team.

Gowns, towels, tools and equipment required for immediate hairdressing treatment must always be readily available for the client when he or she arrives in the salon. This will present a professional image and help save time for you and the stylist. The client then has the treatment completed in good time making the visit a cost-effective one.

Cleaning the work area and sterilising tools and equipment

Remember to clear away all materials, tools and equipment when the stylist has finished with them. Wipe down the styling area with a suitable cleansing liquid at the most appropriate time and make sure the area is hair free. Combs, brushes and all tools and equipment that have come into contact with the client's hair and scalp must be cleaned and sterilised ready for the next client.

CHAT ROOM

Think about how you would feel if a stylist used a comb on your hair that had been used on clients all day without being cleaned and sterilised. Salons are breeding grounds for bacteria. Make sure all equipment is clean for every client.

Methods of sterilisation

Different tools and equipment need to be sterilised using different methods. For example, soft plastics cannot withstand the heat in an autoclave and will change shape (melt!). A plastic roller will come out looking like a chewed piece of gum! Be careful to choose the right method for each piece of equipment. Take advice and guidance from the stylist or senior manager on how to sterilise correctly.

 CHECK IT OUT

❶ Write a list of the different types of sterilisation methods available in your salon.

❷ Find out how each one sterilises. For example, an autoclave will sterilise to 125°C.

What's the difference between sterilising and disinfecting?

Sterilising destroys all living organisms.

Disinfecting an item slows down the growth of bacteria.

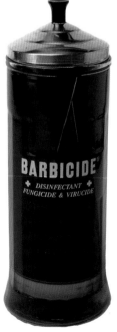

Sterilising solutions and spray

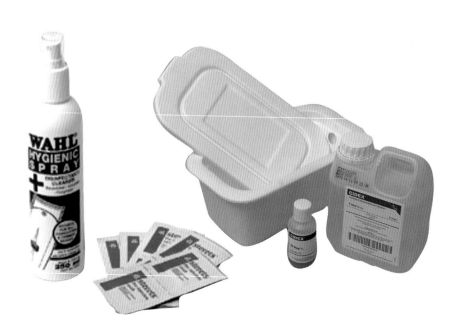

Client records

Record cards are a professional record of what has been applied to the clients' hair. They are a useful tool for recording positive comments and suggestions for any future treatment the client may request.

The personal and professional information contained in record cards is protected by the Data Protection Act (1998) and only professional staff may have access to them for professional purposes. Correct storage of client records in a lockable cabinet is essential to a smooth-running business.

When obtaining records for your stylist's client, remember to check the name, address and telephone number. Clients may share the same surname and even the same initial, particularly if they are from the same family.

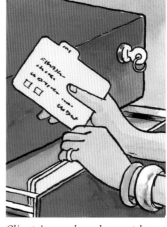

Clients' record cards must be stored in a lockable cabinet

 CHAT ROOM

Clear away and file record cards as soon as they have been completed. Your next client does not want the previous client's colour applied to his or her hair.

Maintain the work area for hairdressing services

Disposing of hair and waste materials safely

The correct disposal of hair and waste materials is vital to the success of the business because the Environmental Health Officer can – and often does – close down salons where staff have failed to deal correctly with salon waste. To remind yourself about the safe removal of waste and materials from the salon, see Unit H1 Shampoo and condition hair.

 CHECK IT OUT

Contact environmental health services at your local authority to find out how to dispose of salon waste in the correct way.

Discuss your findings with your stylist or senior manager.

Control of Substances Hazardous to Health (COSHH) Regulations (2003)

Each local authority has its own policy on how to deal with salon waste. In general, hair should be burned, aerosols should be disposed of separately from the general salon waste and **sharps** should be incinerated.

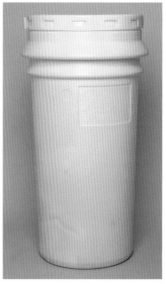

Sharps must be thrown away in a special yellow-coloured bin

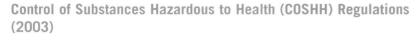

Sharps – *blades used in razors.*

Checking and cleaning equipment

All salon equipment must be checked visually before each use and cleaned after each use in readiness for the next client.

Make sure equipment is cleaned thoroughly following the manufacturers' instructions. Use the most appropriate cleaning materials provided by the stylist or senior manager. Remember to wear suitable personal protective equipment (PPE) when using chemicals or cleaning fluid.

PAT – Portable Appliance Test.

Electrical tools and equipment should be checked by a qualified electrician and **PAT** tested each year. This will satisfy any health and safety checks that your salon may have.

Clean towels and gowns

Checking the appointments at the beginning of every day and throughout the day (appointments can vary) will help you to prepare for each of your stylists.

You will need to find out how many chemical and non-chemical treatments are booked in for the day. Make sure you have clean gowns and towels for every treatment, and always have a ready supply of materials to help the stylist carry out the treatment.

 CHAT ROOM

Sometimes it is a good idea to check the appointments system the day before, especially with chemical treatments. Check you have the necessary perms, relaxers and colours required for each of the clients.

Stock levels

Stock-taking systems vary from salon to salon. It is your responsibility to make sure that no product falls below the minimum stock level. The stylist or senior manager will advise you on how much stock needs to be kept for each product.

Computer systems

Your salon might have a computer system which updates the stock level as you enter sales. The system may also contain clients' records, and details of each stylist's income and retail sales.

CHECK IT OUT

Talk to each member of your team and discuss how it might be possible to improve the stock system. The salon may be happy with its current manual system, but you might be able to suggest a computerised system or maybe a simple system of writing down shortages on a coloured piece of paper. This would need to be kept in a familiar place for all staff to access and complete. Is this something that could be discussed at one of your staff meetings?

Updating information on the computer system could provide you with an opportunity to offer your client something totally different, for example a colour with the cut and blow-dry, or a perm a couple of weeks prior to a holiday. These opportunities make for a better client-stylist relationship.

THINK ABOUT IT

Try to think of a retail incentive scheme where all staff are encouraged to sell retail products and more chemical and non-chemical treatments. This could lead to greater income for the salon and perhaps a higher return for all staff in terms of an increased salary.

Look at the retail chart below and think of a way in which all staff could benefit, from the junior to the senior manager.

| Staff name | SEPTEMBER | | | |
	Week 1	Week 2	Week 3	Week 4
Michelle				Straighteners
Kirsty	Conditioning mousse	Moisturising shampoo	Scrunchie	
Laura		Brush	Serum	
Jelisha	Hair shine		Chemical treatment	

Retail chart – products and treatments sold

At the end of week 4, the salon could simply total the cost of sales and offer an incentive to the member of staff for selling the most. Some hairdressing companies will gladly donate gifts for retail incentives. Discuss this with a senior member of staff and discuss the advantages at your next staff meeting.

CHAT ROOM

Think about all of your clients coming in every day for the coming week. Do you have enough chemical products, shampoos, conditioners, styling products and stock such as hair grips, ornamentation? This part of your work is important, because if you do not have the product, you cannot offer the service.

Cleaning work surfaces

Cleaning work surfaces effectively and leaving them ready for further treatments should include not just the salon itself but the areas where you mix and prepare chemicals and make clients' drinks.

The floor, reception seating area, all working surfaces and mirrors must be kept hygienically clean. Any spillages on the floor must be cleared away immediately. Remember to wear gloves and an apron if necessary.

Floors will need to be swept throughout the day and mopped at the end of each day with a suitable disinfectant. Mirrors will need a suitable glass cleaner to avoid smearing and all working surfaces must be cleaned with a bactericide.

Floors will need to be swept throughout the day

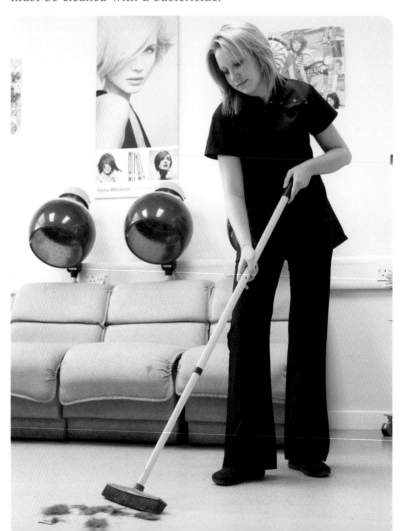

To minimise **cross-infection**, it is essential to follow good housekeeping practices at all times.

Health and safety law requires the salon to keep its refreshments area separate from the area where you mix and dispose of chemical waste. This is essential to good hygiene and a professional standard of working.

> *Cross-infection* – *when an infection (such as a cold) or an infestation (such as head lice) is passed from one person to another.*

 CHAT ROOM

What could be the consequences for a client if you made a drink with bleach powder still inside the cup?

 MEMORY JOGGER

Answer the multiple choice questions below, either on your own or in a small group. There is only one correct answer to each question. When you have finished, check your answers with a senior member of staff.

1 Sterilisation is:
   a the destruction of all living organisms
   b the only method used in salons
   c the least effective method of sterilising
   d the dry method of sterilising

2 An autoclave will:
   a condition the client's hair
   b steam the salon's towels
   c provide a moist method of sterilisation
   d control the growth of bacteria

3 Salon stock should be rotated:
   a to make the shelves look stylish
   b when the salon receives an order
   c every day
   d every month

4 What does COSHH stand for?
   a Control of Substances Hazardous to Health
   b Carried to the Stockroom Hopefully
   c Control of Services to the Salon
   d Control of Stopping Hygiene Problems

5 Salon waste should be:
   a disposed of in a bin
   b disposed of sensibly
   c disposed of in accordance with local bylaws
   d taken home

continued Ⅲ➡

continued ⫘➡

6 Preparing a perm trolley:
   a saves the client time
   b saves salon staff time
   c saves both client and staff time
   d saves time for a lunch hour

7 Cleaning the salon is necessary:
   a to control the growth of bacteria
   b to make it look bright and shiny
   c to comply with health and safety
   d because you may be closed down

8 Client records must:
   a be left on the reception desk
   b handled only by the client
   c locked away safely each day
   d updated only when you feel like it

9 The most recent update to the Data Protection Act is:
   a 1994
   b 1998
   c 2000
   d 2003

10 COSHH was amended in:
   a 1999
   b 2000
   c 2001
   d 2002

One of the most important parts of hairdressing for all clients is shampooing and conditioning.

In this unit you will learn how to:

- maintain effective and safe methods of working when shampooing and conditioning hair
- shampoo and condition hair.

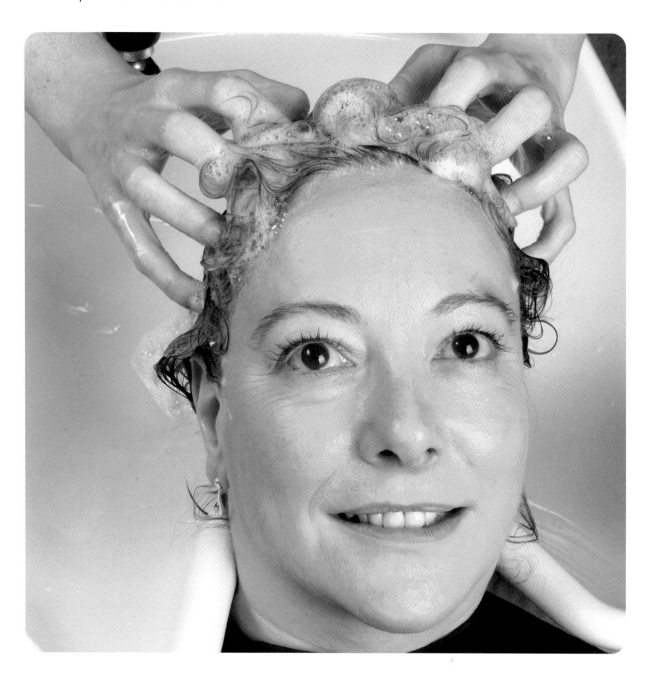

Maintain effective and safe methods of working when shampooing and conditioning hair

Most people can shampoo their own hair at home and are likely to have done so many times. As a practising hairdresser, you will need to make sure that your shampooing technique is of a high professional standard.

Why shampoo hair?

We shampoo hair for three reasons:

- To remove natural oil, skin cells, dust and dirt.
- To remove the build-up of hair-care products.
- To prepare the hair for further treatments.

The success of the shampoo is important to the success of the following treatment, for example the client's cut, perm or colour.

CHECK IT OUT

Look at the various shampoos and conditioners in your salon. Then complete the chart below. The information will be useful when offering clients professional advice about their hair and scalp condition.

Hair/scalp type	Shampoo	Conditioner
Normal		
Dry/damaged		
Fine		
Coloured		
Permed		
Dandruff affected		
Oily		

 CHAT ROOM

Remind clients who are going on a seaside holiday to pack hair-care products such as sunscreen, leave-in conditioner and moisturising shampoo. To help protect the hair, cover it with a sun hat and remove all traces of chlorine and sea water as soon as possible.

How shampoo works

Shampoo comes in many types, consistencies, colours and smells. It mixes with water allowing grease, dirt and oil to be rinsed out of the hair. It contains detergent **molecules**. Each molecule consists of two parts – one part is attracted to dirt and oil, the other part is attracted to water. The tail of the detergent molecule digs into the dirt and oil on the surface of the hair and scalp. The head of the detergent molecule

Molecule – the smallest part that a substance can be divided into.

has a negative **electric charge**. As a result of massage movements, dirt and oil is repelled from the hair and rinsed away in the water.

Water also has a high surface tension that has the effect of producing a 'skin' on the surface of the water. Shampoos flatten the surface tension of water making it easier to shampoo the client's hair.

> **Electric charge** – *a quantity of energy. There are two types of charge – negative and positive. Things with the same electric charge push away from (repel) each other.*

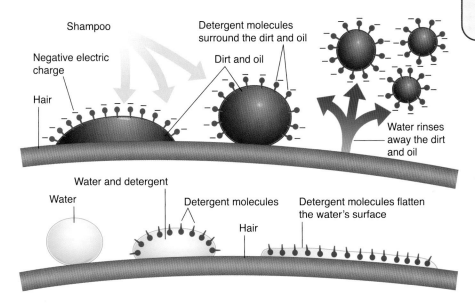

How detergent molecules in shampoo cleanse the hair

Shampoo flattens the surface tension of the water

Conditioners

Hair is made of a protein called keratin. The same protein is found in skin and nails.

Hair in poor condition may have been damaged by overuse of electrical equipment, incorrect brushing or too many chemical treatments. Conditioners strengthen and moisturise the hair.

There are many types of conditioner. They include the following:

- **Surface conditioner** coats the hair shaft and smoothes down the cuticle scales leaving the hair tangle free.
- **Anti-oxidant conditioner** prevents any further oxidation to the hair shaft after chemical treatments.
- **Specialist treatment conditioners** strengthen the hair shaft internally by filling the air spaces caused by damage with liquid protein. This gives the hair added elasticity, sheen and manageability.
- **Almond or olive oils** are used mainly for dry scalps.

 CHAT ROOM

Remind clients who are going abroad to take an adapter for their hand-held hairdryer. They might also like to take a gas-powered styler.

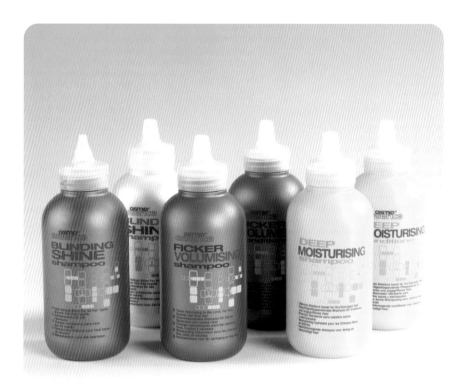

A range of conditioning shampoos

Preparing the client and yourself for the treatment

Your salon's requirements for client preparation should include a thorough hair and scalp analysis by an experienced stylist who will confirm whether it is safe for you to carry out the treatment.

Protecting the client

The client's clothing must be protected at all times. Use a clean protective gown and towel. If the client is not gowned properly during chemical services, his or her clothes may get damaged. The correct client preparation for each service is essential.

 CHAT ROOM

Give clients enough room to breathe when you put a gown on them. Secure the gown with space to tuck a towel in at the collar. Ask clients if they are comfortable.

 CHECK IT OUT

Find out how you prepare the client for the following services:
- Perming.
- Relaxing.
- Colouring.
- Cutting.
- Setting.

Positioning the client and checking your posture

Position the client correctly at either the backwash or frontwash basin and check that he or she is comfortable. The client's position will affect how you stand at the basin and how tired you will feel at the end of the shampoo. Poor posture may have a long-term effect on your wellbeing, so make sure that your position and posture during the shampoo reduce the risk of tiredness and injury to yourself.

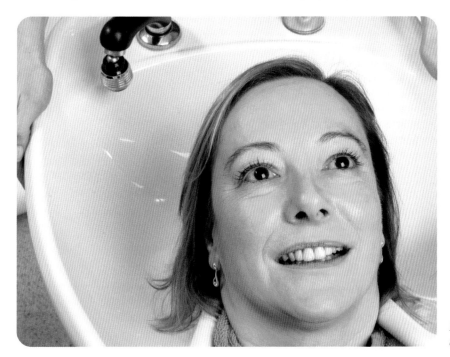

Position the client comfortably at a backwash basin

The work area and removal of waste

Remember to keep your work area clean and tidy at all times.

You will need to remove any waste after each shampooing and conditioning service and dispose of it in a controlled and environmentally friendly way.

Waste to be removed includes:

- loose hair from the frontwash/backwash basin – to prevent blockages
- empty conditioner or shampoo bottles – put these in the salon waste bin
- used tint, bleach and perm lotion – pour these away down the salon basin
- cut hair from the salon floor (to prevent people from slipping) – this should be incinerated (burned) and disposed of by the local authority
- sharp items such as razors – store these in a sharps box (they must be disposed of by a specialist company)
- hairspray, mousse – these must not be incinerated, but be disposed of by a recognised company.

Removing waste promptly and efficiently makes effective use of your time and will give the client a professional image of the salon. It also reduces the risk of injury and cross-infection.

Working methods

Using resources efficiently

Resources such as hairdressing products are expensive and it is important to use them cost effectively. Some shampoos have pump dispensers and these may help to reduce unnecessary waste.

Reducing the risk of cross-infection

All resources that come into contact with clients' skin must be completely clean. This will help to maintain a safe and hygienic working environment. As well as keeping the salon clean, you must always remember your personal cleanliness. Make sure your own standards of health and hygiene reduce the risk of **cross-infection**. For example, do not come into the salon if you have a cold or contagious disease, or infestation such as head lice, as it may cause offence to your clients and colleagues. Stay at home until the condition has cleared and it is safe to return to work.

Cross-infection – when an infection (such as a cold) or infestation (such as head lice) is passed from one person to another.

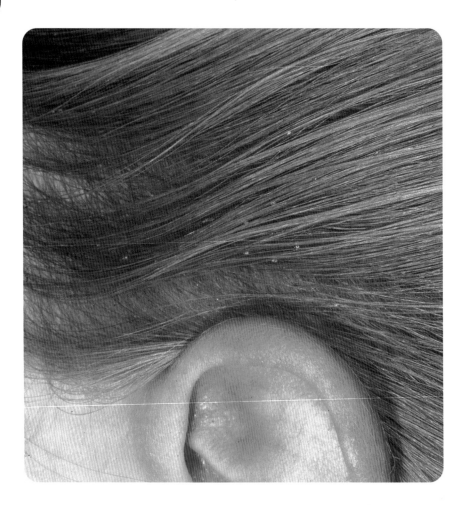

Head lice hatch from eggs called nits. They can be found on the hair shaft close to the scalp

Reducing the risk of injury

Your hands are essential to carry out everyday tasks both in the workplace and at home. If your hands are often in water, you should always dry them thoroughly and use a barrier cream and protective gloves. This will help to reduce the risk of contact dermatitis, a skin condition which often affects hairdressers. It is caused by constant contact with products such as shampoos and chemicals. Should the condition worsen, you should seek medical advice.

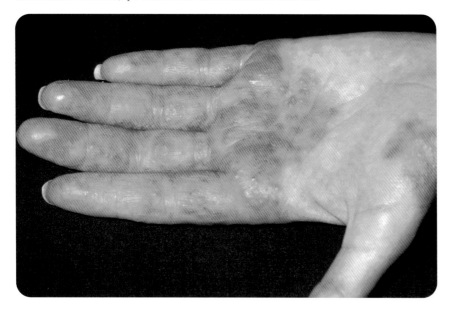

Protect your hands against dermatitis

CHAT ROOM

Leave your rings at home. This will make it easier for you to maintain healthy hands and help prevent dermatitis.

It is essential to store, use, handle and dispose of products in accordance with manufacturers' instructions, salon policy and local bylaws. When dealing with resources in the salon, you will be expected to have a good working knowledge of the Control of Substances Hazardous to Health (COSHH) Regulations (2003) (see Unit G1 Ensure your own actions reduce risks to health and safety). This is for your own and your client's safety.

CHECK IT OUT

1 Whose instructions do you follow when carrying out a shampoo?

2 What may happen if you do not follow the instructions?

3 What problems may arise when carrying out a shampooing and conditioning service? (Think about spillages, water and products.)

Refilling and reordering products

Shampoos, conditioners and chemical products are in constant use in the salon.

 CHECK IT OUT

1 **a** Think of reasons why products need to be reordered and why you will need to keep shampoos and conditioners filled up.

b Who might be disrupted if the salon runs out of a product?

2 Find out who you should report stock shortages to in your salon?

How long should a shampooing and conditioning treatment take?

Depending on the length and thickness of the client's hair, a basic shampoo and surface condition should take 3–5 minutes. You may find it helpful to watch your colleagues and time them.

 CHECK IT OUT

How long does it take you to shampoo a client?

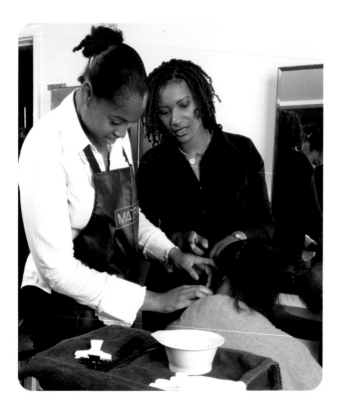

An experienced stylist instructs a junior member of staff

Shampoo and condition hair

Working with the stylist

There are many different levels of staff within the salon, including:

- staff who shampoo and carry out basic skills
- staff who practise technical skills like perming, relaxing, cutting and colouring
- senior staff who may manage the salon.

Part of your job role will involve learning to work with people and take instructions from senior colleagues. They may ask you to use a product in a particular way, or to change your massage movements to suit a different hair type and length.

Using products and tools

Acid and alkali products

Acid and alkali products are regularly used in the salon.

Acid products include perms, colours, shampoos, conditioners, bleach and peroxide. Acid-based conditioners are considered to be kinder to the hair because they close down the cuticle scales and return the **pH** of hair to pH 4.5–5.5. They also maintain moisture within the hair shaft and give a smooth, shiny, tangle-free feel to the hair.

Alkali products include bleach, colours, perms, relaxers and some shampoos. These products lift the cuticle scales and give a roughened feel and appearance to the outer layer of the hair shaft. The pH of the hair is often more than pH 7, which is why the hair must be returned to its natural acid state of pH 4.5–5.5.

> **pH** – *the pH scale measures whether a product is acidic or alkaline, with 1 on the scale being the most acidic and 14 the most alkaline.*

Steamers

A steamer produces a constant amount of steam contained within a hood. The hood is similar to that of a hood hairdryer. It works rather like a kettle. You will use a steamer to help:

* the penetration of the conditioner
* replace lost moisture
* strengthen the internal and external layer of the hair shaft.

You should only use a steamer if you have been trained and know how to use it.

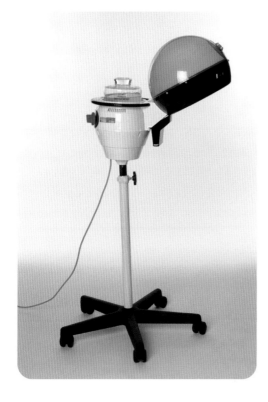

A steamer

The **Electricity at Work Regulations (1989)** cover the safe use of electrical equipment in the salon (see Unit G1 Ensure your own actions reduce risks to health and safety).

First, fill the tiny reservoir with distilled (not tap) water. This is to make sure that no impurities coat the element and block the tiny water valves.

With dry hands, plug in and switch on the steamer. While you massage the client's hair and scalp, the water will heat and produce steam into the hood.

Place the client under the hood for 5–10 minutes. When the timer has switched off, take the client out from the steamer. Switch off and unplug the steamer.

Clean the steamer as soon as you have finished with it, leaving it ready for the next client.

 CHAT ROOM

Offer the client a drink or a magazine to read while under the steamer. Remember the client's care and comfort.

Massage techniques

During the shampoo and application of conditioner, you will need to use certain massage movements. The most popular shampooing and conditioning movements used within the salon are:

- effleurage
- rotary
- petrissage
- friction.

The amount of shampoo you use for each client will be different depending on the length and thickness of the client's hair. A small amount of shampoo, usually no more than the size of a ten pence piece, is usually sufficient. Pour the shampoo into the palm of your hand.

Rub both palms together and then introduce the palms of your hands to the client's hair, smoothing the shampoo down the hair length and on to the scalp.

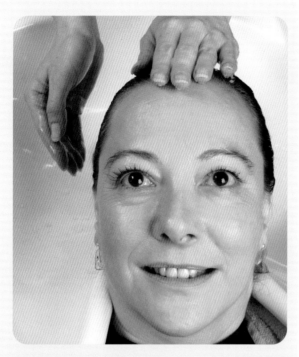

Effleurage movement

Effleurage is used to spread the shampoo throughout the hair at the start of the shampoo and each time you repeat the application of shampoo. Effleurage is a light, slow and superficial movement used as a linking movement to rotary massage.

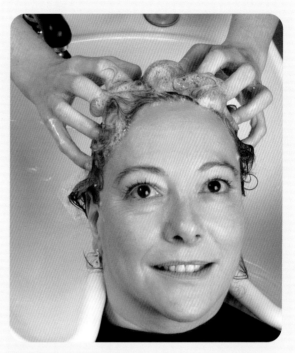

Rotary massage

Rotary massage is used during the shampoo. It is much deeper and faster than effleurage. Your fingers will have a claw-like movement when positioned on the client's scalp with a firm pressure. Small, fast, circular movements are used throughout the scalp when shampooing.

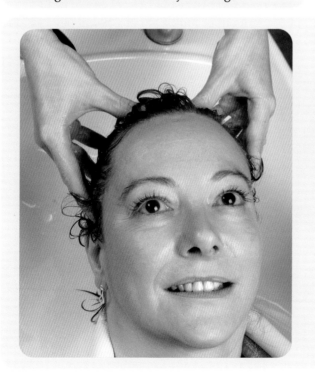

The massage movements effleurage and petrissage are used when carrying out a conditioning treatment. The effleurage movement is used to soothe and calm the client and to introduce the massage movement petrissage.

Petrissage is a slower version of the shampooing movement. It should totally relax the client, assist penetration of the conditioner and promote blood circulation. Petrissage helps to make the hair smooth, shiny and manageable.

Petrissage movements

Friction massage

Friction is a massage movement that involves a fast rubbing technique and has a light, gentle plucking action. It is sometimes used within salons when shampooing or when applying lotions such as astringents.

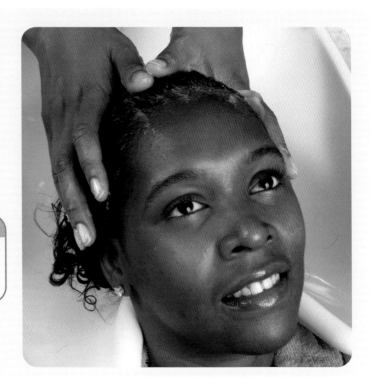

 CHECK IT OUT

Ask a senior member of staff to help you find out what an astringent is used for.

Water temperature and flow

The temperature of the water plays an important part in cleansing the hair and scalp. The flow of water is important too. Both temperature and flow will depend on the amount of hair present and the sensitivity of the client's scalp.

Very hot water may burn the client's scalp, but if the water is not hot enough, the hair will not be fully cleansed. There are times when you may need to use tepid (warm) water. For example, if the client's hair and scalp are oily, tepid water will help the sebaceous glands to produce less sebum when carrying out a lighter massage during the shampoo.

Before and during each shampoo, it is essential to test the temperature of the water, either on the back of the hand or on the inside of the wrist. Remember to check regularly with the client that he or she finds the water temperature comfortable.

Always turn off the tap between shampoos. Hot water is too expensive simply to let it run away!

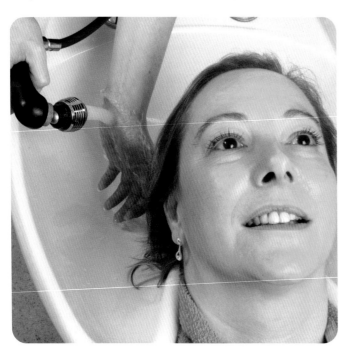

Testing the correct flow and temperature of the water

You will need to choose the most appropriate shampoo for the client's hair and scalp condition. Some treatments that follow a shampoo may not need a conditioner. For example, when perming a client's hair conditioner will coat the cuticle and act as a barrier giving the client an unsatisfactory result.

Be careful not to spill the shampoo, but if you do, you will need to clear up any spillages straight away for the safety of your client, colleagues and yourself.

 CHAT ROOM

Low-soled and low-heeled shoes will help to maintain your posture when you are on your feet all day.

Applying and removing the conditioner

When you have completed the shampoo, you might have to apply surface conditioner using effleurage and petrissage movements. This will smooth down the cuticle scales, maintain moisture levels, protect and promote shine and improve the feel of the hair.

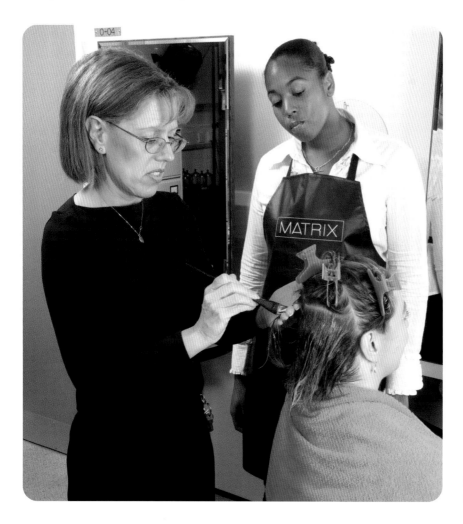

Surface conditioner is applied to protect and promote shine

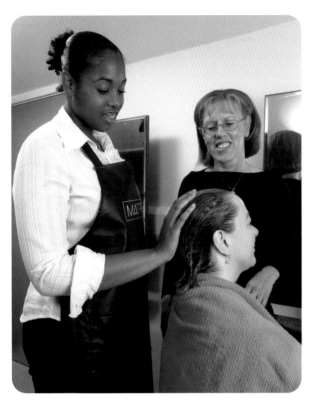

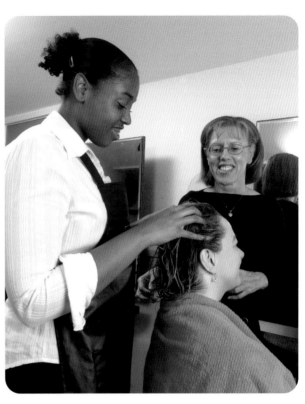

Using effleurage movement when applying conditioner   *Using petrissage movement when applying conditioner*

After you have finished shampooing and conditioning, rinse the hair thoroughly. This is important to the success of the following treatment. Stylists do not want to ask their client to return to the shampoo basin to remove excess product from the hair. Towel-dry the hair and wrap it in a towel, using a turban style.

If you have used a steamer, rinse the client's hair with cooler water than you shampooed with. This will help to smooth down the cuticle scales of the hair ready for styling.

 CHECK IT OUT

Discuss with a colleague the physically harsh and chemically harsh treatments a head of hair may experience. Write a short list.

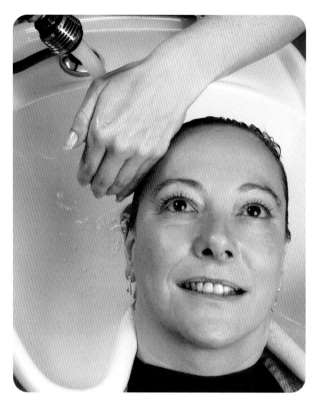

Rinsing the client's hair free of conditioner

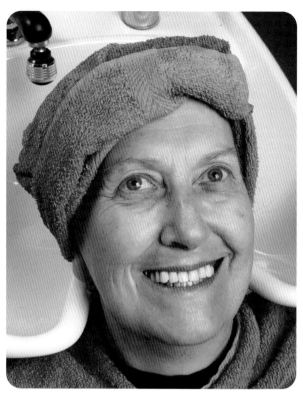

Wrap the client's hair in a towel, using a turban style

Leaving the client's hair free of excess moisture

The stylist will want you to leave the client's hair free of excess moisture and tangle-free. You will need to comb through from the points to the roots of the hair shaft, without causing damage to the hair and scalp, in preparation for the next treatment.

The client will welcome some expert advice and guidance when you discuss how to maintain her nicely conditioned hair at home. Always be knowledgeable about the products your salon retails. Discuss with your client at the consultation stage and at the basin, the suitability of professional shampoo and conditioning products. This will help maintain the moisture level of your client's hair and offer protection in between salon visits.

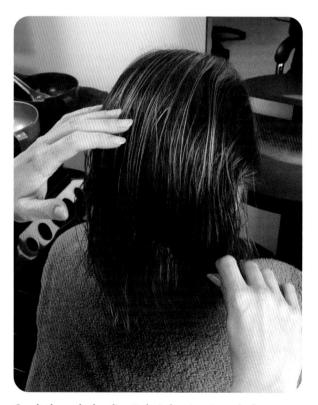

Comb through the client's hair leaving it ready for further treatment

STEP BY STEP

SHAMPOOING AND CONDITIONING

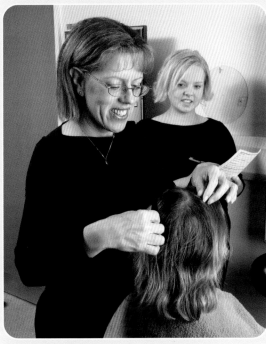

1 Gown up the client and analyse her hair and scalp before shampooing

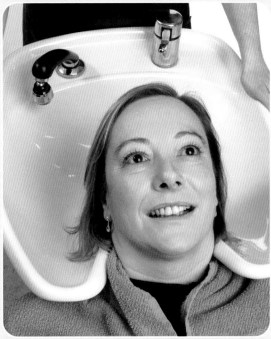

2 Ensure the client is positioned comfortably before shampooing

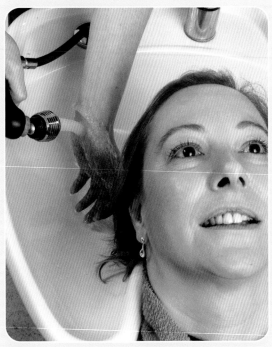

3 Test the temperature of the water before wetting the client's hair

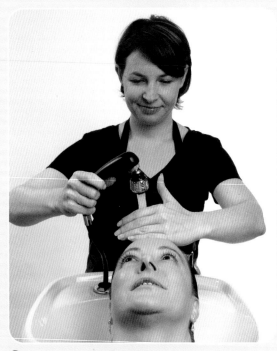

4 Apply the water to the client's hair taking care not to wet her face

STEP BY STEP

SHAMPOOING AND CONDITIONING (CONTINUED)

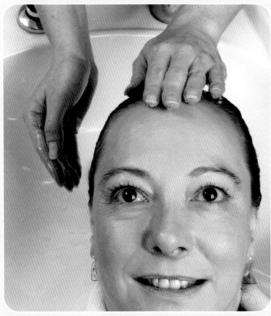

5 Using effleurage movement, apply the shampoo

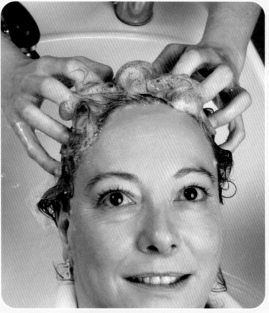

6 Use rotary massage over the whole head until the shampoo lathers and then rinse the hair free from shampoo

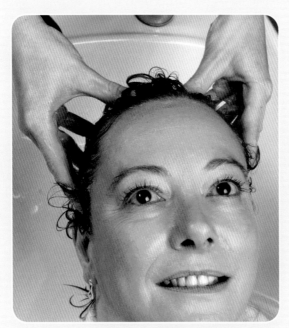

7 Apply the conditioner using both effleurage and petrissage movements. Rinse the conditioner from the hair and turn off the water. Wrap the client's hair in a towel

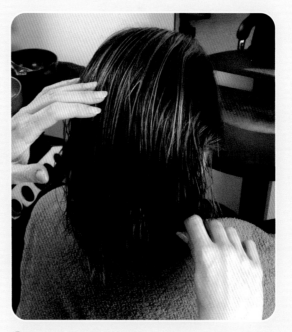

8 Squeeze hair to remove excess water. Place a towel around the client's shoulders to prevent any drips and comb through the client's hair ready for further treatment

MEMORY JOGGER

Discuss the questions below with your colleagues. Then write down your answers.

1. Why must you check salon equipment visually before using it?

2. List and state for what purpose you would use salon equipment.

3. What would you use to clean equipment after each use?

4. Find out where equipment should be safely stored in your salon.

5. Practise your salon's preparation for shampooing and conditioning with a colleague.

6. List the shampoos and conditioners for both European and African-Caribbean hair and scalp types.

7. What are the massage movements used in shampooing and conditioning?

8. Why do we shampoo hair? Give reasons for repeating the shampoo process.

9. Where are spillages most likely to occur in the salon?

10. List three things that should ensure the client is correctly positioned and is comfortable.

11. Why should the water temperature and flow be checked when shampooing?

12. What are your responsibilities under COSHH (2002) Regulations?

In this unit you will be assisting the stylist with the basic skills of perming, relaxing and neutralising.

Perming is the chemical process of curling hair by permanently altering its structure. Relaxing is the chemical process of straightening naturally curly hair. Neutralising is the chemical process that fixes hair into its new shape after it has been permed.

You will learn about removing colouring and lightening products from the hair and materials such as foils, easi meche and the highlighting cap.

Chemical treatments for European and African-Caribbean hair types are slightly different and you will need to be able to work with both.

In this unit you will learn how to:

- maintain effective and safe methods of working when assisting with perming, relaxing and colouring services
- neutralise hair as part of the perming and relaxing processes
- remove colouring and lightening products.

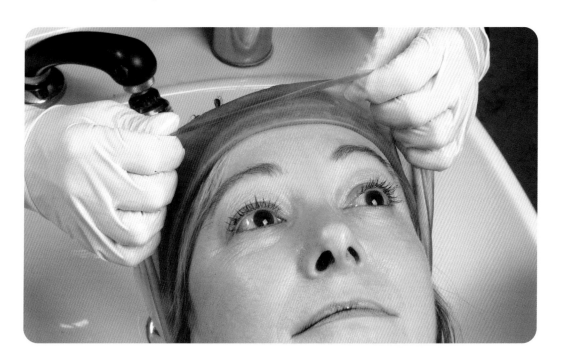

What makes hair straight or curly?

What makes hair naturally straight or naturally curly? One suggestion is that the shape of the follicle determines the shape of the hair shaft. Another suggestion is that straight hair has a circular cross-section and curly hair has an oval cross-section.

Altering straight or curly hair

Hair may be straightened temporarily using heated styling equipment. This is a very popular salon treatment, but one that needs careful handling because repeated use of styling equipment can damage the hair.

 CHECK IT OUT

List the different types of styling equipment that can be used to produce a straight effect on the hair.

Keratin – a protein from which hair, nails and skin are made.

The straightness or curliness of hair may be permanently altered by treating the hair with a suitable chemical treatment. This produces a permanent change in the structure of **keratin**. When the natural structure of the hair is changed chemically, the disulphide bonds in the cortex layer of the hair shaft are altered.

Because the change is permanent, it can only be removed by cutting or growing the hair out, or reversing the treatment chemically.

Great care must be taken when using chemicals on clients' hair as overprocessing will damage both the internal and external structure of the hair.

Acid and alkaline perms

Acid or alkaline perms can be used on the client's hair, depending on the result required. Before choosing the perm, the stylist must consider the condition and type of hair that is being treated.

Acid perm lotions may be used on hair that is already dry, damaged or porous where strong alkaline perm lotions might cause breakage.

 CHECK IT OUT

What types of perm lotion are used in your salon for different hair types and conditions? Discuss this with your senior stylist.

Perming hair

There are two main stages to perming hair.

Stage 1 Breaking down the hair's disulphide bonds

During this stage the disulphide bonds are broken down to take on the shape of the rod that is being used. This stage is carefully timed to make sure that the correct amount of bonds is broken.

If the hair is overprocessed, there is a risk that it will break. If it is underprocessed, the curl result may be unsatisfactory. The manufacturer's instructions and your stylist will tell you exactly how long to leave the perm lotion on the hair before rinsing.

Stage 2 Fixing the hair into its new position – neutralising

In this stage you will be asked to rinse the hair thoroughly for a certain period of time. Usually a minimum of five minutes is needed to flush out the perm lotion from the hair.

After you have rinsed the hair, you will need to blot out the excess moisture before applying a neutraliser containing hydrogen peroxide or sodium bromate. The neutraliser is an **oxidising agent** which helps to re-form the disulphide bonds broken down by the perm and fixes the hair into its new position.

> Oxidising agent –
> adds oxygen to the hair.

Correct timing of the neutralising process is crucial to the finished result. Overprocessing can leave the hair frizzy and underprocessing will give a weak curl result.

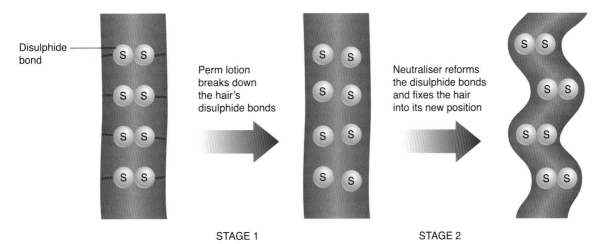

Disulphide bond

Perm lotion breaks down the hair's disulphide bonds

Neutraliser reforms the disulphide bonds and fixes the hair into its new position

STAGE 1

STAGE 2

The two stages of perming

Maintain effective and safe methods of working when assisting with perming, relaxing and colouring services

Protecting the client's clothing

This is where you put into practice everything you have learned in earlier units. Your client must be protected with suitable waterproof capes, gowns and clean towels.

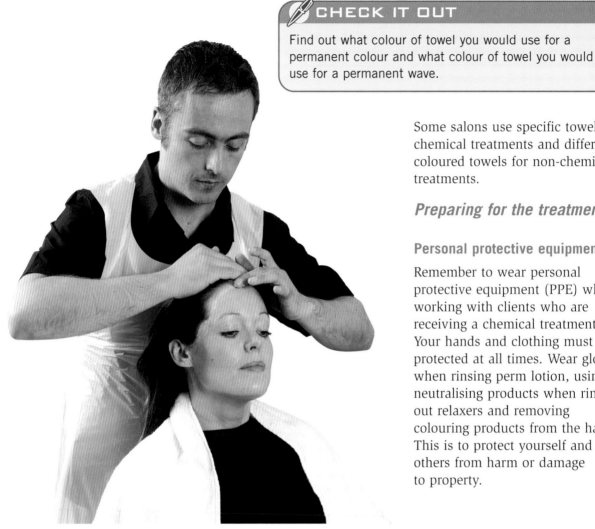

Always wear personal protective equipment when carrying out a chemical treatment

CHECK IT OUT

Find out what colour of towel you would use for a permanent colour and what colour of towel you would use for a permanent wave.

Some salons use specific towels for chemical treatments and different coloured towels for non-chemical treatments.

Preparing for the treatment

Personal protective equipment

Remember to wear personal protective equipment (PPE) when working with clients who are receiving a chemical treatment. Your hands and clothing must be protected at all times. Wear gloves when rinsing perm lotion, using neutralising products when rinsing out relaxers and removing colouring products from the hair. This is to protect yourself and others from harm or damage to property.

Resources

RESOURCES FOR PERMING AND RELAXING

- Trolley
- Selection of combs
- Plastic bowl
- Cotton wool
- Apron
- Gloves
- Section clips
- Tension strips
- Client's record card
- Barrier cream
- Plastic cap*
- Additional heat source for perming – climazone*
- Rods
- End papers
- Towels
- Gown

* These items may be needed

You may need to assist the stylist by passing up perm rods and end papers.

RESOURCES FOR COLOURING AND LIGHTENING

- Clean towels of the appropriate colour
- Hydrogen peroxide (sometimes)
- Foils
- Easi meche
- Highlighting cap
- Tinting bowl and tinting brush
- Record card

- Colour trolley
- Gown
- Cape
- Barrier cream
- Cotton wool
- Shade chart

All resources must be hygienically cleaned after every use. For example, do not mix bleach with a tint brush that has been used for applying a raspberry grape tint. Using clean tint brushes, combs, section clips, gowns and towels will help to minimise the risk of cross-infection.

Preparing the client for shampooing

Before shampooing, you will need to comb through the client's hair. Remove tangles carefully to avoid causing the client any discomfort. Check the client's scalp with the stylist, looking for any cuts or areas that may need special attention. You will also need to discuss with the stylist the correct shampoo to use.

Positioning the client and checking your own posture

As you prepare the client for shampooing, discuss with the client whether he or she prefers a frontwash or backwash basin. Position the client at the basin taking care to make sure he or she is comfortable. The client's comfort and also your position and posture when using the basin are important to minimise the risk of injury and fatigue both to yourself and the client. During shampooing the client may be splashed with water, so it is a good idea to offer the client a towel to safeguard against unavoidable splashes.

Positioning the client and yourself correctly is once again important as you carry out the neutralising process. Check with the client his or her choice of a frontwash or a backwash basin. If the client requests a backwash, make sure that the client's neck is positioned into the curve of the basin, otherwise the nape area may not be neutralised properly which could result in an unsatisfactory result and could also be uncomfortable for the client.

The pre-perm shampoo

The pre-perm shampoo will remove the build-up of hair-care products, open the cuticles and leave the hair in a neutral **pH** ready for either an acid or alkaline perm lotion. Pre-perm shampoo has a neutral pH value of 7.

Note: Do not shampoo hair before using a relaxer as this will open pores and the relaxer may burn.

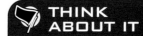
THINK ABOUT IT

In error, you use a tint brush which was used previously to apply a rich red colour, but had not been washed out properly, for bleaching. What would happen to the client's hair colour?

pH – the pH scale measures whether a product is acidic or alkaline, with 1 on the scale being the most acidic, 7 being neutral and 14 the most alkaline. Hair is acidic and has a pH of 4.5–5.5.

STEP BY STEP

THE PERMING PROCESS

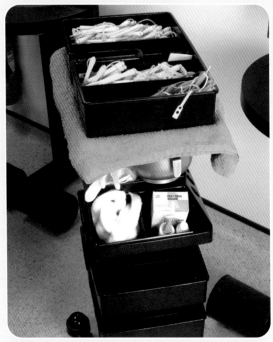

❶ Ensure the trolley is prepared prior to perming

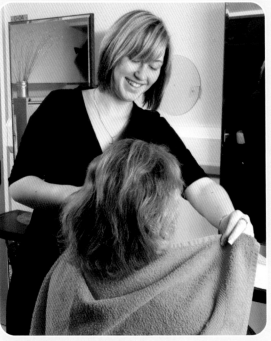

❷ Gown the client for a perm

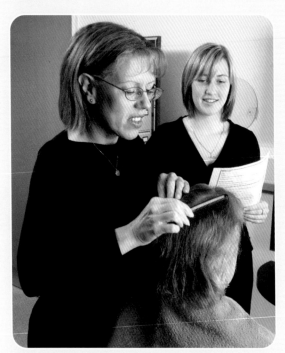

❸ Carry out a hair, skin and scalp analysis on the hair by dividing the hair into sections

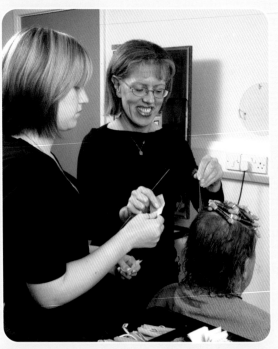

❹ Pass rods and papers to the stylist as she needs them

STEP BY STEP

THE RELAXING PROCESS

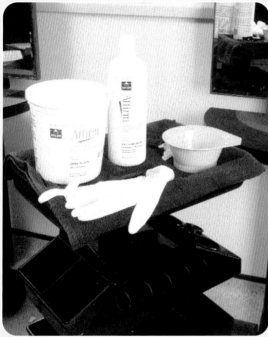

1 Ensure the relaxing trolley is prepared prior to treatment

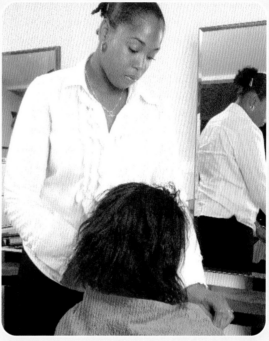

2 Gown the client for relaxing

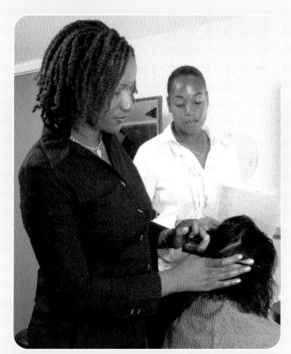

3 Carry out a hair, skin and scalp analysis on dry hair by dividing the hair into sections

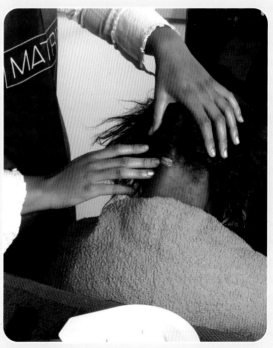

4 Apply barrier cream to the hairline taking care not to apply it to the hair

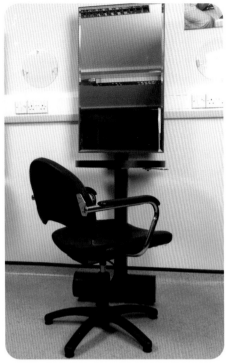

The work area should be kept clean and tidy

Keeping your work area clean and tidy

It is essential to keep your work area clean and tidy during chemical treatments. Position tools and equipment for ease of use and prepare the basin area ready for use. This will help to ensure that all tools, equipment and materials are readily available and provides an efficient method of working during the treatment.

Working safely

Working with chemicals

Before using chemicals, always read the manufacturer's instructions and discuss them with the stylist. If you are asked to mix a chemical product, remember to mix only the amount that you need just before it is to be used.

Some manufacturers advise using scales to weigh the product for an accurate mixture. This will help to reduce wastage. If extra mixture is required, it is more cost-effective to make it fresh. It is also an effective use of your time.

Vitality
Vita Perm
Permanent wave

Instructions for use (Read thoroughly)

1 Preparation:
- Check the condition and porosity of the hair then select the correct lotion.
- Shampoo the hair using a mild shampoo. Rinse thoroughly and towel dry.
- To equalise hair porosity for an even curl result, a pre-perm treatment is recommended.
- Section the hair and select appropriate curler size for the chosen technique, then wind without lotion. Vitality End Papers make winding easier.

2 Application:
- Wear protective gloves.
- Carefully apply the perm lotion onto each curler, using the applicator nozzle.
- Repeat if necessary to ensure thorough penetration, but do not over-saturate.
- Allow to develop

3 Development guidelines:
The suggested development times in the guidelines overleaf have been tested thoroughly and produce optimum results. However, if you are unsure about the overall condition and porosity of the hair, we recommend that test curls should be taken to determine the final development time. Development times can be increased as required but care should be taken to avoid over-processing. When correct curl strength is achieved, rinse hair thoroughly for 5 minutes.

4 Rinsing and Neutralising:
After completion of development time rinse all curlers thoroughly (2–3 minutes). Thoroughly blot the curlers to remove excess moisture.

Foam neutraliser
- Pour 50ml of the neutraliser into a non-metallic bowl.
- Add an equal amount of warm water.
- The neutraliser is now ready to use.
- For maximum neutralisation, use a neutraliser sponge and apply two thirds of the neutraliser evenly to all the curlers, foam up thoroughly (do not foam up in the bowl).
- Leave to develop for 5 minutes.
- Gently unwind all the curlers and apply remaining one third of the neutraliser through the hair.
- Distribute evenly and allow to develop for a further 5 minutes.
- Rinse thoroughly.
- Blot out excess moisture with a clean towel.

5 After care
After rinsing out we recommend the use of a suitable after-care treatment.

Vitality UK Ltd. Newtown NW1 1AB

Manufacturer's instructions for a perming treatment

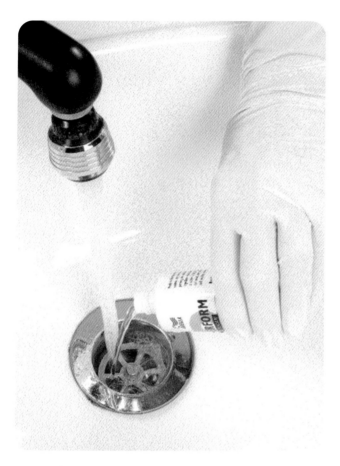

Chemical waste should be flushed down the shampoo basin

CHECK IT OUT

1 With the help of a stylist, carry out an incompatibility test. You will need:
- a non-metallic bowl
- scissors
- a sample of hair
- hydrogen peroxide
- perm lotion.

2 Ask your stylist about other types of hair and scalp tests that you need to know about, for example skin test, pre-perm test curl, development test curl, porosity test and elasticity test.

Disposal of chemicals

Always flush waste tint, hydrogen peroxide, neutraliser, relaxer and perm lotion down the shampoo basin, followed by lots of cool water to make sure no smells linger round the basin. Some salons may have a specific basin for disposing of hazardous chemicals safely.

The Control of Substances Hazardous to Health (COSHH) Regulations require you to dispose of waste products safely in accordance with the manufacturers' instructions, salon policy and local bylaws. Never pour chemicals down the salon's kitchen sink, especially if this is where you wash and dry clients' cups and saucers.

Checking for hazards and risks

Always keep a look out for hazards or risks which may arise during the course of the day. Clear away used product bottles, used tint bowls or neutralising sponges and cotton wool. Keep the floor clear from trailing cables, towels, gowns, cut hair and shopping bags or children's buggies. This will help to minimise the risk of harm or injury to yourself and clients.

Carrying out an incompatibility test before perming

The stylist may want to carry out an incompatibility test to make sure that the client's hair is suitable to perm. Some previous treatments may react badly when perm lotion and neutraliser are applied.

For example, metallic salts which are found in hair colour restorers and compound henna may cause the hair to boil, bubble and break. If metallic salts are suspected, the stylist will not perm the client's hair.

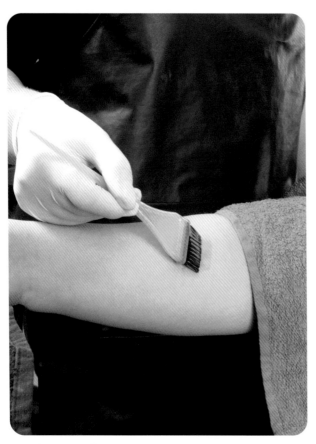

Carrying out a skin test

Always write down the results of tests you carry out on clients on their record card. This will give the salon a record of what you have done and give the client confidence that the results of any test are recorded for professional purposes. Store the record card once it has been completed by the stylist and possibly by yourself in a record card box (for information on data protection, see Unit G2 Assist with salon reception duties).

Carrying out a skin test before colouring

All clients must have a skin test 24–48 hours before colour is applied. This includes semi-permanent colours, quasi colours, permanent colours and may also include vegetable colours.

If the instructions are not followed, the consequences could be serious. It may result in damage to the hair and scalp and even chemical burns should the wrong type of heat be applied to the hair for further processing. Always work with great care when dealing with chemicals.

A natural colour such as a vegetable colour may be a suitable alternative to an oxidation tint. They are unlikely to cause dermatitis and do not usually require a skin test. Remember, not all clients can use natural products on their skin, so it is worth checking if the product is suitable. The timing of processing may require the addition of oxygen from the atmosphere so the final colour result will not be achieved until the next day.

 CHECK IT OUT

Test some hair samples with different types of colour.
Note down how different the condition of the hair is and
how vibrant the shades of colour are.

Taking care of the client

Offer the client drinks and magazines at appropriate times. The best time is usually while the client's chemical treatment is processing.

Personal health and hygiene

Remember to practise good personal hygiene and wear clean, well-pressed clothes (see Unit G1 Ensure your own actions reduce risks to health and safety).

Any sign of personal infection or infestation must be reported straight away to a senior member of staff in order to minimise the risk of cross-infection and offence to clients and colleagues.

 CHAT ROOM

If you run out of a product which needs reordering, remember to follow salon policy and write it down or tell the appropriate member of staff.

This will make sure that you have sufficient products available for use and avoid having too much stock.

Neutralise hair as part of the perming process

Neutralising the client's hair re-forms the disulphide bonds and fixes the hair structure into the shape of the perm rod being used.

 CHECK IT OUT

Find out how to prepare the neutraliser that your salon uses by first reading the manufacturer's instructions and then discussing them with a senior member of staff. Talk about your findings with a junior colleague.

Rinsing out the perm lotion

You will need to follow both the stylist's and manufacturer's instructions when rinsing the client's hair free from perm lotion. At the end of the processing time, the hair should be rinsed for a minimum of five minutes to thoroughly remove all traces of perm lotion. It is best to use warm water – the client should find this comfortable – which will leave the cuticles of the hair open, enabling the neutraliser to penetrate more effectively.

Towel blotting the hair

The hair must be free from excess water before the neutraliser is applied. To remove excess moisture, you will need to towel-blot the hair. It is worth taking time to do this properly as too much water in the hair will dilute the neutraliser and ruin the perm. Check how wet the hair is by placing your hands over the client's rods – if you find lots of water on your hand, you must continue with towel blotting. Some salons may use tissue or cotton wool to remove excess water from the client's hair.

STEP BY STEP

NEUTRALISE EUROPEAN HAIR AS PART OF THE PERMING PROCESS: STAGE 1

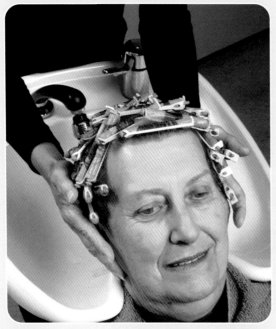

① Position the client at the basin and rinse hair thoroughly

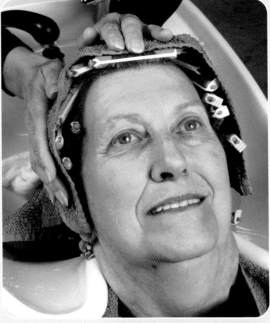

② Towel-blot the hair to remove excess water

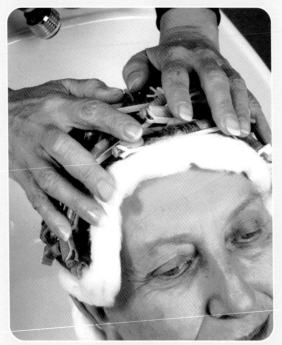

③ Check any remaining excess water by passing your hands over the client's rods

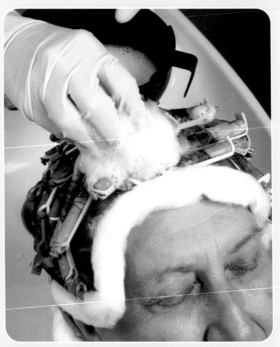

④ Apply the neutraliser to each rod and allow to process according to the manufacturer's instructions

STEP BY STEP

NEUTRALISE AFRICAN-CARIBBEAN HAIR AS PART OF THE PERMING PROCESS: STAGE 1

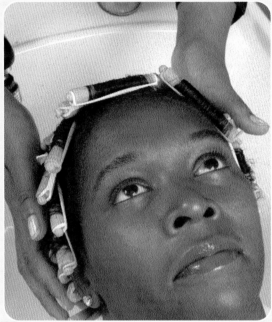

❶ Position the client at the basin and rinse the hair thoroughly

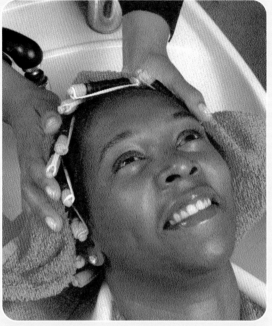

❷ Towel-blot the hair to remove excess water

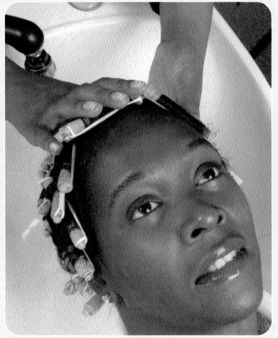

❸ Check any remaining excess water by passing your hands over the client's rods

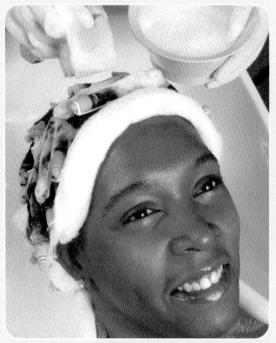

❹ Apply the neutraliser to each rod and allow to process according to the manufacturer's instructions

Preparing the hair for neutralising

■ Wear gloves and a suitable apron to prepare the neutraliser.

■ Protect the client's skin with barrier cream and damp cotton wool around the hairline – this will help protect the skin around the hairline from any chemical damage which may be caused by the neutraliser.

■ Using either dry cotton wool or a clean dry towel, carefully blot each perm rod to remove excess water.

■ Promptly refer any concerns or problems to the stylist or senior manager to find out the course of action to take.

Using the neutraliser

There are two main types of neutraliser used in the salon:

■ hydrogen peroxide neutralisers

■ sodium bromate neutralisers.

Some neutralising products can be used straight from the bottle, others will need preparing by foaming up the product in a bowl. The stylist will instruct you on how to use a particular product. You should also read the manufacturer's instructions which will explain how to use the neutraliser safely and effectively.

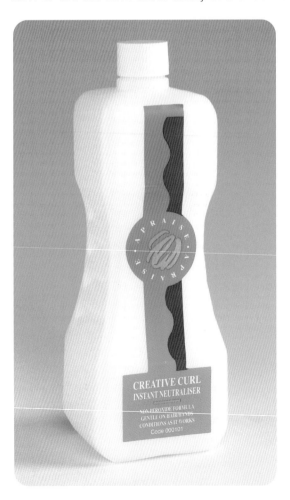

Neutralising products for European hair

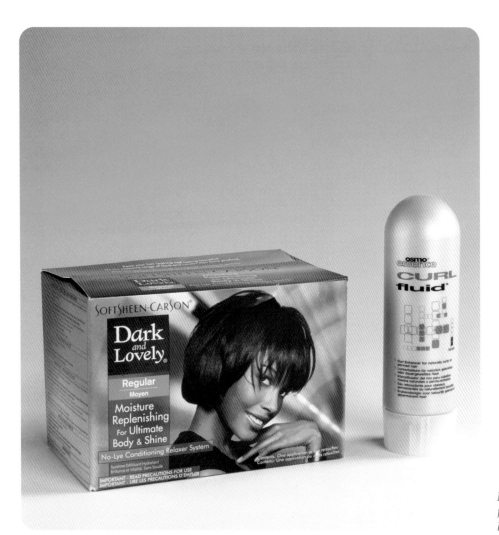

Neutralising products for African-Caribbean hair

You must match the correct neutraliser with the perm lotion being used. For example, an alkaline perm must be followed through with a hydrogen peroxide neutraliser. This is because sodium bromate reacts explosively with ammonium thioglycollate, an ingredient of alkaline perm lotions. Sodium bromate is effective with acid perm lotions and can also be found in neutralisers suitable for African-Caribbean hair as the chemical minimises hair discolouration.

Applying the neutraliser

Apply the neutraliser following the manufacturer's instructions, but first confirm with the stylist that you know exactly how to do this. Make sure that you apply the neutraliser evenly throughout the client's wound hair. Take care when applying lotions, for example you will need to consider the client's position and comfort. Avoid any area which has not been permed. This hair can be protected by using gel or conditioner on the hair that has not been wound.

Removing the rods

Remove the rods carefully without disturbing the curl formation. The hair is in a very delicate state at this stage. Rough handling may cause scalp irritation or damage, including making the hair straight.

Some neutralisers will instruct you to keep the rods in during the neutralising process, while others will ask you to remove the rods after approximately five minutes before continuing with the second part of the process. Always follow the manufacturer's instructions and confirm with the stylist what you should do.

 CHAT ROOM

Neutralisers used on African-Caribbean hair contain sodium bromate, a gentler chemical than hydrogen peroxide. Sodium bromate neutralisers take longer to fix the new curl pattern which is why the rods remain in the hair throughout the neutralising process.

Removing all the neutraliser

Rinse off the neutraliser thoroughly so that no traces are left on the hair. This will prevent chemical damage to the hair and makes sure the new shape is fixed.

Timing the neutralising process

It is essential to time the neutralising process accurately. The disulphide bonds in the cortex of the hair shaft need a certain amount of time to re-form. Overprocessing or underprocessing will give a poor result. You may find it helpful to use a timer to accurately time the processing. Some types and lengths of hair may need a longer time to develop depending on the amount of hair that has been wound around the rod.

Perming and neutralising problems

Problems may occur if instructions are not followed correctly or the wrong products are used. The hair could be left in a fragile state, for example it may return to its straight natural look if the neutraliser is left on too long, the product may cause damage to the scalp leaving the skin irritable and broken, there may be discolouration, frizziness, uneven curl along the hair length, or straight hair at the sides or at the nape area of the scalp.

Mistakes and problems can and do happen! When they do, stay calm, and refer to the senior stylist immediately. To reduce the risk of problems, always check each stage of the procedure with the stylist before you start. The chart below shows some of the more common perming and neutralising problems and how to deal with them.

Fault	Correction	By whom	How to avoid
Fish hooks	Remove by cutting	Stylist	Cover points of hair with end papers
Overprocessing	Cut and condition	Stylist/junior	Carefully time the process using the salon clock or timer. Record the processing time on the client's record card
Neutraliser applied unevenly	Re-perm if the condition of hair allows	Stylist	Check the stylist's/manufacturer's instructions. Monitor application of neutraliser.
Skin and scalp irritation	Rinse immediately with cool water	Junior	Appropriate test before chemical treatment
Hair breakage	Cut to disguise and use restructurant to strengthen hair	Stylist	Pre-perm/incompatibility test

Perming and neutralising problems and how to correct them

Applying conditioner

Remove excess moisture from the client's hair by squeezing out the water by hand. Then apply a suitable anti-oxidant conditoner to the client's hair. Leave the conditioner on the hair for at least three minutes.

Anti-oxidant conditioners will:

- replace lost moisture
- help prevent further oxidation of the hair
- return the pH of the hair to its normal acid value.

Remove the conditioner following the manufacturer's and stylist's instructions. Towel dry the client's hair and wrap it in a turban style before taking the client to the styling area. Clean and tidy the basin area making sure that all used products are disposed of correctly, leaving the area free from risk, hazard, cross-infection or infestation.

STEP BY STEP

NEUTRALISE EUROPEAN HAIR AS PART OF THE PERMING PROCESS: STAGE 2

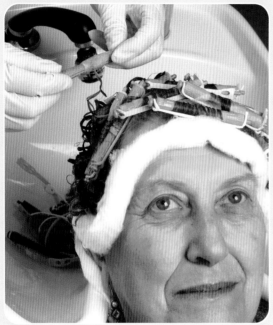

5 Remove the rods and rinse thoroughly to remove all traces of neutraliser

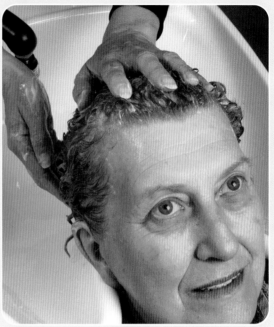

6 Apply conditioner to the hair

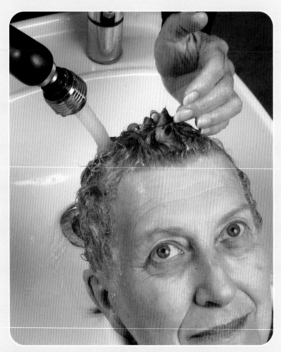

7 Rinse the conditioner from the hair

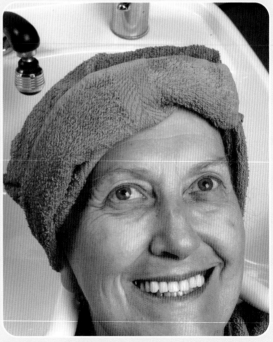

8 Towel dry the hair and then wrap it in a turban style ready for styling

STEP BY STEP

NEUTRALISE AFRICAN-CARIBBEAN HAIR AS PART OF THE PERMING PROCESS: STAGE 2

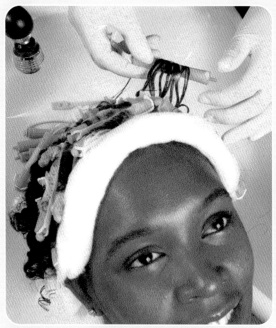

5 Remove the rods and rinse thoroughly to remove all traces of neutraliser

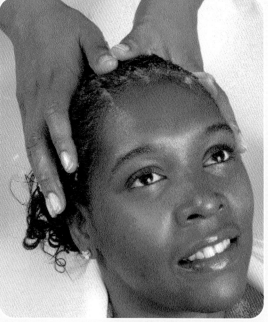

6 Apply conditioner to the hair

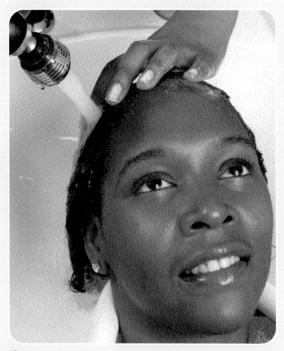

7 Rinse the conditioner from the hair

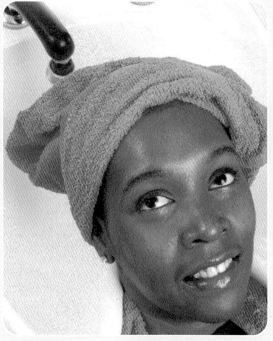

8 Towel dry the hair and then wrap it in a turban style ready for further styling

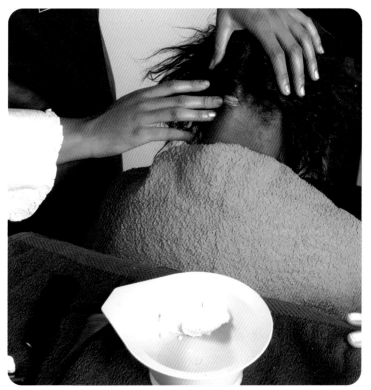

Application of barrier cream prior to relaxing

Neutralise hair as part of a relaxer service

Prior to relaxing, a protective base or barrier cream should be applied to the scalp, which is easily removed when the hair is shampooed after the relaxing process.

Pre-relaxer treatments

Pre-relaxer treatments are used on hair that is very porous. They coat the cuticle with a polymer film which acts as a barrier to slow down the action of the chemical product. They should be used on the middle lengths of the hair.

CHAT ROOM

- Never apply relaxer to wet hair as this could cause breakage.
- Apply a protective base to the scalp before carrying out the relaxing process.
- Do not offer the client a hot drink before or during the relaxing service. It could make the client hot which would cause the relaxer to develop too quickly and the scalp may become irritable.

Using a neutralising shampoo

Once you have rinsed the relaxer thoroughly from the hair, you should use a neutralising shampoo to make sure the hair is free of relaxer. The neutraliser will rejoin the disulphide bonds in the cortex layer of the hair shaft. After shampooing the hair (at least three times), towel dry the hair and apply conditioner.

CHAT ROOM

- Always use gloves when rinsing and neutralising.
- Do not massage or rub the scalp vigorously when rinsing out relaxer. This could irritate the scalp.
- Check hair is free from relaxer before applying post-perm treatment.

Applying a post-perm treatment

The next stage is to apply a post-perm treatment which will leave the hair in a manageable condition. These products are acidic and will bring the hair back to its normal pH level and moisturise the hair after the chemical relaxing process.

CHAT ROOM

- Not all product manufacturers produce a post-perm treatment. Some offer a product that can be used across a range of relaxers.
- Follow the stylist's and manufacturer's instructions when using post-perm treatments.

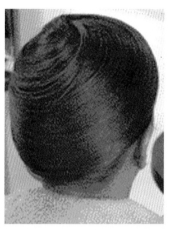

The finished result of relaxing

Remove colouring and lightening products

Colouring and lightening are chemical treatments which will be offered within your salon.

Using only a hint of colour can alter the appearance of the client. Many clients are introduced to the world of hair colour by trying out temporary colours. These are fun to use and can be applied to dry or wet hair in minutes.

CHAT ROOM

You could try to interest clients in temporary colours by wearing a suitable colour in your own hair. Try different coloured hair mascaras, coloured sprays, coloured mousse, coloured setting lotion, glitters and coloured gels.

Other clients may prefer a colour from the semi-permanent range. This will give them time to think over the advantages of a permanent colour.

CHAT ROOM

Not everyone would want pink highlights in their blonde hair. Colour selection is important. Remember, temporary colours may stain bedclothes.

What gives hair its colour?

Is it black, brown, red or blonde? Hair gets its colour from colour-giving cells known as melanocytes. These are found in the **dermis** layer of the skin and are produced in the cortex of the hair shaft. Melanocytes produce either eumelanin or pheomelanin. Eumelanin gives black or brown **pigment** and pheomelanin gives red and yellow pigments.

Dermis – *the inner layer of the skin.*

Pigment – *a substance that colours something.*

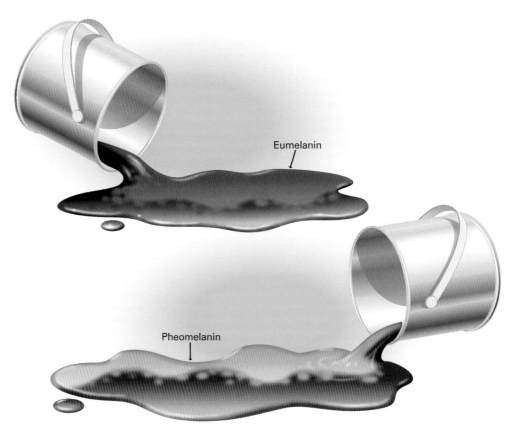

Eumelanin

Pheomelanin

Different combinations of pigments in the cortex produce many different natural colours and shades of hair. Where a person has no pigments in the hair shaft, he or she will have white hair – this is due to the melanocytes no longer producing colour pigment. Reasons for white hair include ageing, hereditary, trauma, shock, stress or childbirth.

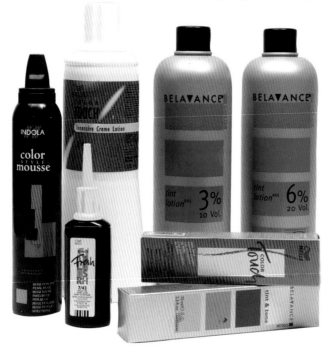

A range of colouring products

Colouring products

Your salon may stock the following colouring products:

- temporary colours
- semi-permanent colours
- quasi colours
- permanent colours
- lightening products
- vegetable colours.

CHECK IT OUT

With a colleague, find out:
a the different types of colouring and lightening
   products available within your salon
b how they are applied
c how long they last on the hair.

Salon and legal requirements

Client preparation for colouring and lightening treatments varies from salon to salon.

If the stylist has chosen a colour that needs a skin test, then this must be carried out before you continue with the treatment. The result of any test must be recorded on the client's record card.

Once the stylist agrees that it is safe to proceed, consult with the client and observe how the stylist prepares the client for a colouring treatment. You will need to assist by combing the client's hair and checking for cuts and areas that need special attention.

Colouring problems

When removing colouring products and materials such as foils, easi meche or a highlighting cap, they must be taken out of the hair in such a way that minimises the risk of damage to the hair. Always remember to follow the stylist's and manufacturer's instructions. You will have your own limits of authority when dealing with problems that may arise during the removal of colouring products.

The types of problems you may come across include:

- colour bleeding on to an area of hair that has not been coloured
- bleach splashing into a client's eyes
- ripped hair – caused by the highlighting cap being removed roughly, which may also cause the client discomfort
- an unsatisfactory result – caused by easi meche or foils being removed before the end of the processing time.

Removing hair colouring materials carefully will minimise the risk of colour being spread to the client's skin, clothing and surrounding areas of the hair.

The chart below shows some common colouring problems and how to deal with them.

Fault	Correction	By whom	How to avoid
Colour seepage	Apply barrier cream to hair that has not been coloured	Stylist	Prepare the client before application of the chemical treatment
Bleach in client's eyes	Rinse with cool water immediately	Stylist	Careful removal of colouring materials and products
Vigorous removal of of the highlighting cap	Condition hair/massage scalp	Junior	Apply conditioner on to the cap prior to removal
Hair colour too warm	Apply toner	Consult stylist	Check base shade and use correct strength of products

Colouring problems and how to correct them

Remember to dispose of all chemical waste down the salon basin followed by plenty of cool water to make sure that no smells linger around the basin. This may include hydrogen peroxide, bleach and colour.

CHECK IT OUT

Discuss the limits of your authority with the senior stylist and find out what you can and cannot do should you meet a problem.

CHAT ROOM

Check out the types of lighting in your salon. Do you have fluorescent tubes, spot lights or incandescent lights? Try encouraging your manager to go green and install fluorescent bulbs. They use up to 75 per cent less electricity and last nearly ten times as long.

Removing colouring and lightening products

Before removing colouring or lightening products, check with the stylist and make sure you read and follow the manufacturer's instructions. Some products require you to **emulsify** the colour before water is applied to the hair and scalp. This is important as the colour will not come off the skin if you miss this simple step.

Emulsify – *using the colouring product to help in removing itself by moving the finger pads around the client's hairline.*

Should there be any problems, refer them to the relevant person – usually the stylist – for the best course of action.

Applying surface conditioner

Once the colouring or lightening product is removed, you may have to use a colour removal shampoo. Squeeze out the excess moisture from the hair, then apply a suitable anti-oxidant conditioner or surface conditioner. Check with your stylist which conditioner to use. (Look back to page 81 to remind yourself what an anti-oxidant conditioner does.)

 CHAT ROOM

Encourage your salon to go green if it isn't already! Use cool or warm water when washing salon towels. The bills will be lower and the salon's energy usage will be more efficient.

Rinsing the client's hair and preparing for the next treatment

Towel dry the client's hair and scalp and make sure that both hair and scalp are clean and free from excess products and moisture. Take the client to the styling area for further treatments and comb through the client's hair, leaving it tangle-free and without damaging the hair or scalp. Both stylist and client need to be satisfied that you have removed all products from the client's hair.

After care

It is important to explain to clients how they should look after their hair at home. After-colour care involves helping the client to maintain the colour of his or hair at home using the most appropriate shampoo and conditioner for colour-treated hair. This is part of professional client care, and by selling the client the correct products, you will be giving him or her expert advice and guidance which completes the colouring treatment.

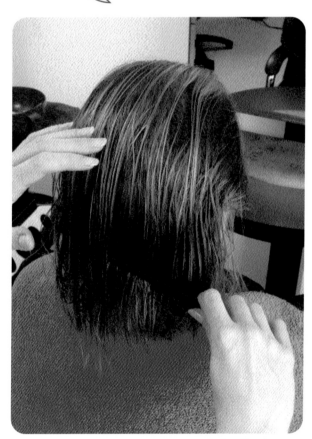

Comb through the client's hair to make sure it is tangle-free, ready for further styling

 CHAT ROOM

Red heads have more hair than brunettes. Brunettes have more hair than blondes.

STEP BY STEP

THE COLOURING PROCESS

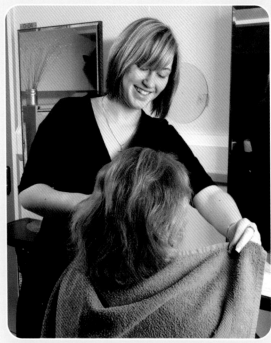

1 Gown the client for colouring and prepare the trolley

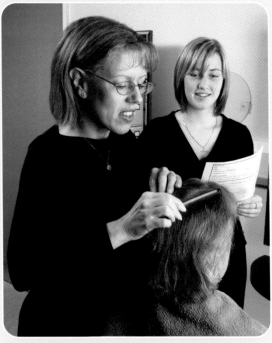

2 Prepare the client for colouring. This involves hair and scalp analysis, and combing and sectioning dry hair

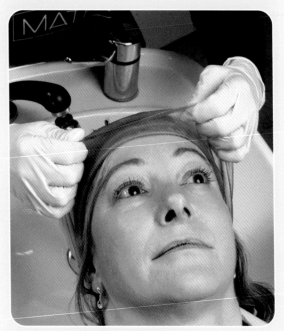

3 Remove colouring products

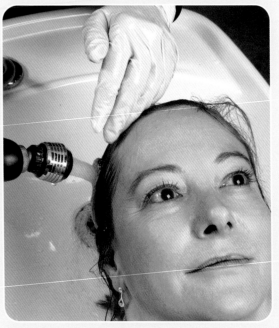

4 Rinse the hair

MEMORY JOGGER

1 What might be the cause of:
   a perm rods falling out during neutralising
   b skin or scalp irritation
   c client discomfort?

2 What might happen if you do not follow the stylist's or manufacturer's instructions?

3 Give reasons why you should follow the stylist's instructions.

4 State what your salon's procedure is for each of the following:
   a handling and storing tools
   b disposal of waste.

5 Who would you report each of the following problems to:
   a client discomfort
   b colour stains around the hairline
   c straight pieces of hair around the sides and nape area
   d products still in the hair after rinsing?

6 Why should you wear personal protective equipment?

7 What would you do if you noticed a stock shortage?

8 List two safety considerations when neutralising.

9 Why should tools and equipment be positioned for ease of use?

10 Why should work areas be left clean and tidy?

11 Why should the client be gowned and protected?

12 Why should you rinse the hair thoroughly?

13 What may happen if you do not use the correct neutraliser?

14 How should you dispose of excess perm lotion?

15 If you have a problem who should you report it to?

16 Which bonds are broken when perming the hair?

17 In which layer of the hair shaft does perm lotion change the structure?

Index

Bold page numbers indicate illustrations.